Christine McMillan-Bodell

HAIRDRESSING & BARBERING

3rd edition

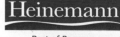

Heinemann is an imprint of Pearson Education Limited, a company incorporated in England and Wales, having its registered office at Edinburgh Gate, Harlow, Essex, CM20 2JE. Registered company number: 872828

www.heinemann.co.uk

Heinemann is a registered trademark of Pearson Education Limited

Text © Christine McMillan-Bodell, 2009

First published 2009

12 11 10
10 9 8 7 6 5 4 3

British Library Cataloguing in Publication Data
A catalogue record for this book is available from the British Library.

ISBN 978 0 435468 30 9

Edited by Rachael Williams
Designed by Wooden Ark
Typeset by Tek-Art
Original illustrations © Pearson Education Ltd, 2009
Illustrated by Mark Watkinson
Cover design by Wooden Ark
Picture research by Caitlin Swain
Cover photo/illustration © Anne Veck Salon, photographer Marco Loumiet
Printed in Spain by Graficas Estella

Websites
The websites used in this book were correct and up-to-date at the time of publication. It is essential for tutors to preview each website before using it in class so as to ensure that the URL is still accurate, relevant and appropriate. We suggest that tutors bookmark useful websites and consider enabling students to access them through the school/college intranet.

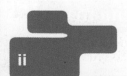

Contents

Acknowledgements

The author and publisher would like to thank the following individuals and organisations for permission to reproduce photographs: Anne Veck/Marco Loumiet p6; Masterfile/Robert Karpa p8; Alamy Images/PlainPicture GMBH&co.KG p19(bottom left [BL]); Science Photo Library/Cordelia Molloy p19(bottom right); Carlton Professional p29(BL), 173(BL); iStockPhoto/Greg Nicholas p34; Image by TONI&GUY p38, 84, 104; Anne Veck/Clark Wiseman p54, 72, 158; Image Source p68, 144; Goldwell p69; Science Photo Library p88, 89; Denman p109(combs); HairTools p109(crimping irons); Anne Veck/Julian Knight p118, 132; GettyImages/Giulio Marcocchi p155(bottom), 160; Anne Veck p166(image 1), 168; JG photography/Alamy p171; Biophoto Associates/Science Photo Library p172(bottom). **All other photos:** Pearson Education Ltd/Mind Studio; Pearson Education Ltd/Gareth Boden/Chris Honeywell/Jules Selmes/Tudor Photography.

For their invaluable help and expertise at the Level 1 photoshoot the author and publisher wish to thank Anne Veck of Anne Veck Salons and the staff at her Bicester location. Thanks are also due to our models, Alice Carter and Catherine Lewis.

Every effort has been made to contact copyright holders of material reproduced in this book. Any omissions will be rectified in subsequent printings if notice is given to the publishers.

Author acknowledgements

Updating this book has enabled me to meet some truly professional people who are committed to hairdressing and care about it deeply as a vocation. When faced with challenges in life, it can be easy to put things off. But with planning and a positive attitude it is surprising what can be achieved. So often I use the words, 'I can, I am and I have.' Hard work and a lot of give and take is what you need to put in as you approach a long and rewarding career in hairdressing. Good luck to each of you!

Without the never-ending love, support and commitment of my family and friends, this book certainly would never have been written. I would like to dedicate this book to my partner Neil who has recently been diagnosed with head and neck cancer – he has always given 110% support.

Thank you to Banbury Postiche of Oxfordshire for their help, Anne Veck Hair Design, Bicester for her expertise and thank you to our models. Finally, to all at Heinemann (publishers, editors, artists, researchers): thank you.

Foreword by Andrew Barton

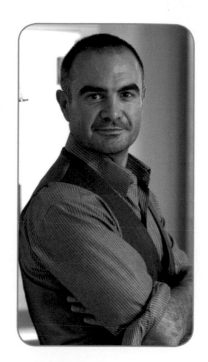

For a working class lad from a small town in Yorkshire, I've not done too badly. I've recently been named the most expensive and sought after hairdresser in the UK – pretty impressive to think that I started in a village salon! For me, there is no such thing as a typical day. One day I'm working with celebrities on a glamorous photo shoot, the next I could be travelling the world flying the British hairdressing flag with Saks at glitzy hair shows and educational seminars. I'm also recognised as TV's favourite hair expert and love spending time making clients happy at the Saks flagship salon in London. So how did all this come about?

I started a very traditional hairdressing apprenticeship in my home town of Barnsley in Yorkshire, which was tough and very disciplined, but years later I'm forever grateful for it. Along with attending college to study for my hairdressing qualifications, it was the best possible start. Learning all the key skills to the best standard has undoubtedly helped me further down the line in my career at Saks. Whether it's been working on everyday clients, supermodels, superstars or creating hair for super designers at the catwalk shows, it's always important to have a good foundation of knowledge.

When I was at the first stages of my career, I had to remind myself constantly to be patient and know that I could not learn everything at once. Keeping a diary of what I learned really helped me to see just how far I had come.

I think I have the best job in the world and I'm amazed by just how much excitement I get from my work every day. Working with a great team is possibly the best advice I can offer anyone. Never accept an OK standard and push your own creativity through experimentation and trial and error.

Hairdressing is competitive, it's fast, ever-changing and of course it's about providing a service, and the service of making someone feel great about themselves through their hair is wonderful. I swear, the smile a client shows you on her face when you've done her hair is magical and addictive!

Because hairdressing is always changing, there's always something to learn and discover, whether new products or techniques. You'll never be bored and as British hairdressing and training are widely acknowledged as the best in the world you're guaranteed to have the best start for the career of your dreams!

Andrew Barton x

Andrew Barton
Saks International Creative Director
www.saks.co.uk

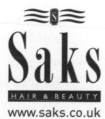

Saks
HAIR & BEAUTY
www.saks.co.uk

Introduction

Why choose a career in hairdressing?

Hairdressing is a multi-billion pound industry and employs approximately 200,000 people in the UK. As hairdressing is constantly evolving, creative people are always needed to meet the demands of an ever-changing industry.

Today's hairdressers cater for the needs of a multi-ethnic society: from European to Asian and African type hair, there is a growing demand for skilled hairdressers. A vast range of products and resources, including the latest organic treatments, are available to you as a hairdresser and to your clients, helping you make an informed choice of the most appropriate treatment for your client.

Combining realistic work experience with developing your knowledge and understanding makes for a level-headed approach to achieving a professional qualification. Once you are a hairdresser, there is an exciting future waiting for you in a high-tech industry, with the chance for you to become your own boss or consider other routes such as image consultant, sales representative, teaching, wig-making, salon manager, freelance hairdresser, specialist hairdresser, colour technician, perm technician – whatever you choose to do. Wherever you go, people will always need their hair to be styled, so enjoy your job security and travel the world!

About this book

This book will take you through the basics of hairdressing and barbering. It covers all of the relevant performance criteria and range statements linked to the latest National Occupational Standards required to complete the Level I qualification in Hairdressing and Barbering.

European and Asian hairdressing is the main focus of the book. It includes the latest units in barbering, blow-drying, plaits and twists and hair extensions, with illustrated step by step guides to help you learn a variety of practical hairdressing procedures. The introductory unit, All about hair, covers what you will need to know about the basic structure of hair and the different hair types.

The book is divided into two sections.

- In the workplace contains all the units which relate to your work with clients and colleagues, as well as your responsibilities in the salon.

- Practical skills deals with the practical hairdressing procedures you need to learn.

To help you achieve each unit of work, the book contains:

» Get up and go! features designed to involve you in an active role in your learning and development

✂ Sharpen up! features that will help you think about the practicalities of hairdressing and the type of situations you will have to deal with every day

? Memory jogger features for you to test your knowledge so you know what you might have to brush up on

⬆ Get ahead features designed to help you make the step from Level I through to Level 2, preparing you for the world of work which lies ahead.

What is an NVQ/SVQ?

A National Vocational Qualification (NVQ) or in Scotland a Scottish Vocational Qualification (SVQ) is made up of separate units that set out exactly what you must be able to do, and to what standard. The diagram below shows how the qualification is structured. If you are doing this qualification with City & Guilds it is called a Level I Diploma.

The practical work you carry out will be linked to the performance criteria in each unit, and the assessor will mark you against the standards set by the awarding body. This means you must carry out certain practical activities to the standard set out by the awarding body, and your assessor will help you with this.

Level I Hairdressing and Barbering consists of **four** mandatory units plus **two** optional units. To achieve the full qualification you need to achieve **six** units in total.

The following units are **mandatory** and must be completed:

- G20 Make sure your own actions reduce risks to health and safety
- G3 Contribute to the development of effective working relationships
- GH3 Prepare for hair services and maintain work areas
- GHI Shampoo and condition hair

You must also complete **two** of the following optional units:

- G2 Assist with salon reception duties
- GH2 Blow-dry hair
- GH4 Assist with hair colouring services
- GH5 Assist with perming hair services
- GH6 Plait and twist hair using basic techniques
- GH7 Remove hair extensions
- GBI Assist with shaving services

All about hair

What is hair?

Hair is made up of a protein called keratin. Your skin and nails are made from the same protein. A strand of hair is called a hair shaft, and it is made up of three layers: the cuticle, cortex and medulla.

Hair structure

The hair shaft is covered in overlapping cuticles, which can be thought of as being like fish scales or the tiles on a roof. When the hair is in good condition, the cuticles lie flat and when the hair is in bad condition the cuticles may be lifted or even torn away, exposing the cortex layer of the hair shaft.

Hair in good condition

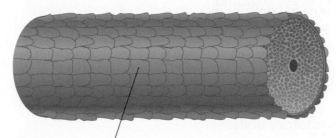

Cuticle scales lying close together

Hair in bad condition

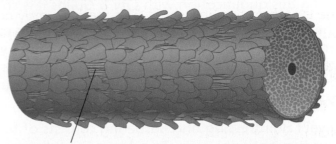

Cuticle scales open and misshapen. Some scale may have been completely destroyed, exposing the cortex

> Hair in good and bad condition

The effect of humidity on the hair is dependent on how well conditioned the hair shaft is and how flat, smooth and even the cuticle scales are. Hair is 'hygroscopic', which means that it absorbs moisture from the atmosphere. Hair that is porous will absorb moisture from the atmosphere more readily than hair that is non-porous. You should take great care when working on porous hair so as not to over-dry it. Directing airflow down the length of the hair shafts can help protect the cuticles.

≫ Get up and go!

Look at some different types of blow-drying products and consider their purposes. Think about products which can be used before and after the blow-dry. Create a chart of styling products and list the most suitable types of hair to use them on and what effects they will have. Show this information to your stylist or assessor and discuss the benefits of each product.

Cuticle

The outer layer is known as the cuticle layer of the hair shaft. The cuticle has overlapping scales wrapped around the centre of the hair known as the cortex. The hair when in good condition reflects the light and is smooth and shiny. The cuticle scales will also be tightly compacted giving a non-porous outer layer.

Cortex

The cortex layer of the hair shaft is made up of bundles of fibrils. Imagine a bundle of dried spaghetti or a bundle of pencils in your hand and this will reasonably reflect the structure of the cortex layer of the hair shaft. In the cortex we can see chemical changes altering the basic structure of the hair shaft. For example, when we perm the client's hair or apply a permanent colour we alter the basic structure of the hair. All chemical changes take place in the cortex. This includes bleaching, relaxing, permanent colouring and perming.

Medulla

The central layer of the hair is known as the medulla. It has no part to play in hairdressing treatments; it is simply made up of air spaces along the length of the hair shaft. The medulla may be present in some hairs but not in others, and may not be present for the full length of the hair.

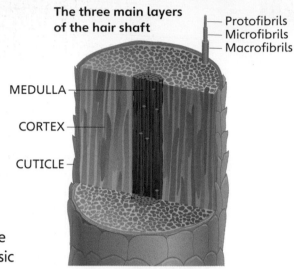

The three main layers of the hair shaft

- Protofibrils
- Microfibrils
- Macrofibrils

MEDULLA
CORTEX
CUTICLE

The hair shaft

Why do we have hair?

Protection

Hair has a protective function. If an object were to fall on your head the hair on your scalp would offer some, although limited, protection. The hair inside your nose acts as a filter when breathing, helping prevent dust and debris from entering your nasal passages, and your eyelashes offer some protection against dust entering your eyes.

Warmth

Hair acts as an insulator by helping keep the surface of the skin warm. You may notice when you are cold that hairs will stand up. This is the body's attempt to keep warm, by trapping a layer of warm air between the surface of the skin and the hair, which is standing up.

Looking good

How does your hair make you feel? Mostly when our hair looks good, we feel good! Hair offers a different dimension to how we feel about ourselves and how we can express ourselves. A freshly shampooed and well conditioned head of hair will give us an added confidence when compared with a head of hair which is greasy and in need of some tender loving care. Growth patterns of the hair may affect our choices of style, and you will need to consider the root direction of a client's hair when helping them select a style.

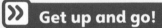
Different face shapes

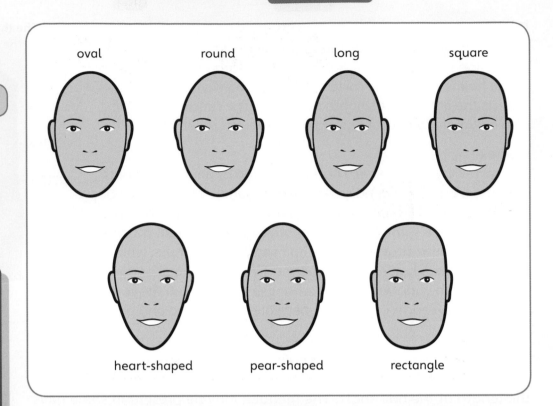

oval   round   long   square

heart-shaped   pear-shaped   rectangle

» Get up and go!

You are what you eat! As you have learned, hair is made up of a protein called keratin, and the basic building blocks of proteins are amino acids. We get these amino acids from the foods we eat, so you really can affect the condition of your hair with the types of food you eat. Think about the food you eat and the effect it might have on your hair. Hair loss and scalp problems can be caused by a poor diet and if our diet is poor, the likelihood is our hair will suffer.

Keep a food diary for one week, keeping a note of the food you eat and its nutritional value. Do you think you are getting enough protein, carbohydrates, vitamins and minerals to feed your body and your hair?

Your hair acts as frame around your face, rather like a frame around a painting. And your hair can be styled to complement your face shape and to disguise less attractive features. Think about a client who may have a very wide forehead; would you give them a fringe?

Hair condition and hair types

Hair and scalp conditions can be divided into dry, normal, greasy and dandruff-affected.

Hair in good condition is soft to touch and hair in bad condition feels rough, dry and brittle. Hair can also be one of the following different types:

- Caucasian/European
- Asian/Oriental
- African type.

You will notice the hair is either straight or has an amount of natural wave or curl present.

- The Caucasian/European hair shaft can be straight, wavy or curly and its cross-section is oval shaped.
- The Asian/Oriental hair shaft can be straight and/or coarse and its cross-section is round.
- The African type hair shaft can be tightly or loosely curled and its cross-section is kidney shaped.

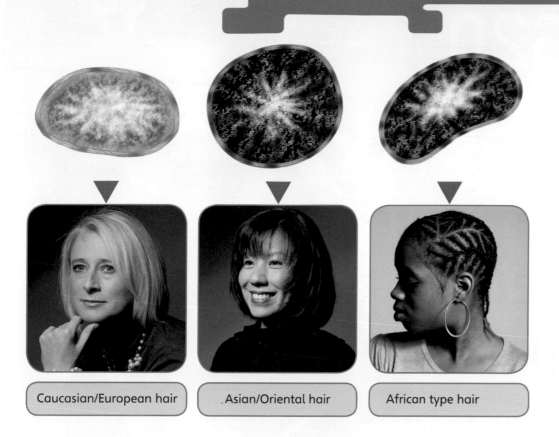

| Caucasian/European hair | Asian/Oriental hair | African type hair |

The texture of hair will vary from client to client and may also vary within the same head of hair. Texture can be fine, medium or coarse and is determined by touch.

Get ahead

Research the hair growth cycle as part of your preparation towards Level 2. Consider the follicle and how it widens at the bottom to encompass the papilla. Find out about the epidermal cells and how these are constantly growing and being pushed up towards the surface of the skin. Write a small project using the following headings and ask your assessor to look at it.

- Alpha and beta keratin
- How the cells change shape as they move along the hair follicle
- The cuticle, cortex and medulla
- Colour producing cells (melanocytes)
- The three stages of the hair growth cycle: anagen, catagen and telogen

Include photos and sketches to help the reader understand what you are explaining.

? Memory jogger

What protein is hair made of?

Name the three layers of the hair shaft.

What happens to the cuticles when hair is in either good or bad condition?

Where in the hair does chemical change take place during certain hairdressing services?

Why do we have hair?

Name the three different hair types and describe how they differ.

UNIT G20

Make sure your own actions reduce risks to health and safety

Anne Veck, photographer: Marco Loumiet

Hairdressing is a fun-loving, people-oriented industry, but to stay safe you need to follow certain procedures when you are using electrical equipment and chemicals and when working with the public. Continual training is essential to reduce accidents and the occurrence of poor health and environmental damage in the salon. With the necessary training, you will be a more effective and successful hairdresser – would you go back to a stylist who used dirty brushes in an untidy and neglected salon, no matter how brilliant the cut and colour?

Health and safety covers three key areas: your responsibility to your clients; your employer's responsibilities to you, your colleagues, clients and visitors; and your responsibility to your colleagues and yourself.

You need to be aware of the risks in your workplace and how to deal with them. This will help you ensure that your actions do not create any health and safety hazards and that you do not ignore hazards that present risks in your workplace. You must take responsible action to resolve things, including reporting situations which may present a danger to people in your workplace, and seeking advice.

In this unit you will learn about:

- Identifying the hazards and evaluating the risks in your workplace
- Health and safety laws
- Workplace policies
- Personal presentation and behaviour
- Safe working practices.

Here are some key words you will meet in this unit:

Job description – a detailed description of the specific duties you must carry out

Workplace responsibilities – rules and regulations you must abide by

Equipment – items such as hairdryers, steamers, ultraviolet cabinet, scissors

Precautions – a preventative measure to safeguard your health and safety

Alert – to be watchful for anything that needs to be attended to

Reporting – a system for alerting other people to a situation

Personal presentation – how you present yourself for your day to day work

Products – the products you use on an everyday basis, e.g. shampoos, colours, perm lotion

Cross-infection – an infection which can transfer from one person to another

Professional image – the high standards of a professional place of work, e.g. current and relevant salon equipment with well trained staff

Environment – the working environment must be a healthy and safe place to be

Instructions – a detailed list of how to carry out a treatment or how to use a particular product

Controlling risks – measures which are put into place to prevent a risk escalating

Safe working practices – working practices which show your method of work is safe and without risk of harm

Additional assistance – help from a colleague or other resource

Identifying the hazards and evaluating the risks in your workplace (I)

This unit covers the health and safety duties for everyone in the hairdressing industry. Every employee and employer is required to behave safely and professionally. You must always be responsible for your own behaviour and make sure your actions do not create a health and safety risk. For example, if you see something in the salon which is potentially dangerous you must take sensible action towards putting things right. This may involve writing the risk down and/or reporting it to a more senior member of staff.

Hazards, risks and control

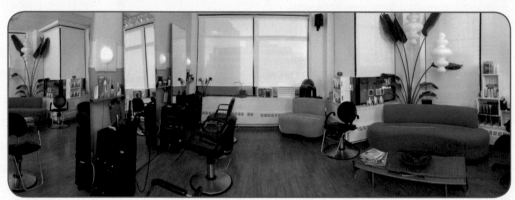

The salon is a great place to work. However, you must be aware of risks and hazards

It is extremely important you understand the terms 'hazard', 'risk' and 'control'. The Health & Safety Executive (HSE) is the body appointed to support and enforce health and safety laws. They have defined the terms listed above in the following ways:

- hazard – something with potential to cause harm
- risk – the likelihood of the hazard's potential being realised
- control – the means by which risks identified are eliminated or reduced to acceptable levels.

Almost anything may be a hazard, but may or may not become a risk. You need to demonstrate you understand the health and safety requirements and policies in the salon. You should be constantly improving your own working practices and work areas, preventing any risk of you or others being harmed. You must be able to identify risks arising from any hazards you have identified. You must know which hazards you can deal with safely in accordance with workplace instructions and legal requirements. Work within the limits of your own authority and report any situation you feel needs the attention of a more senior member of staff.

Sharpen up!

Evidence is important when creating your portfolio. You must provide examples of how you have taken steps to reduce health and safety risks.

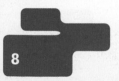

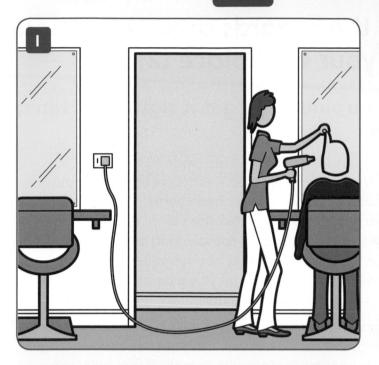

A trailing electrical cable is a hazard. If it is laying across a walkway there is a high risk of someone tripping over it, but if it lies flat to the floor alongside the wall out of the way, the risk is much less.

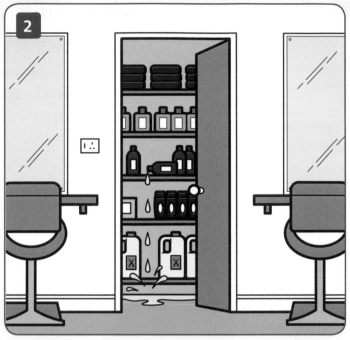

Poisonous or flammable chemicals are hazards and may present a high risk. However, if they are kept in a properly designed secure store and handled by professionally trained people, the risk is much less than if they are left out in the salon for anyone to use – or misuse.

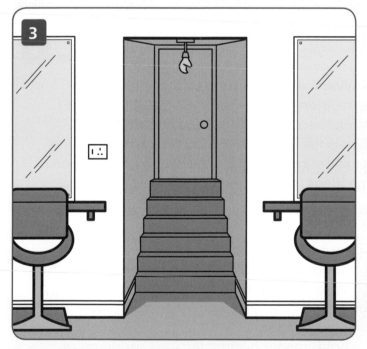

A failed light bulb is a hazard. If it is just one bulb out of many in a room, it presents very little risk, but if it is the only light on a staircase, it is a very high risk. Changing the bulb may be a high risk if it is high up, or if the power has been left on, or low risk if it is in a table lamp which has been unplugged.

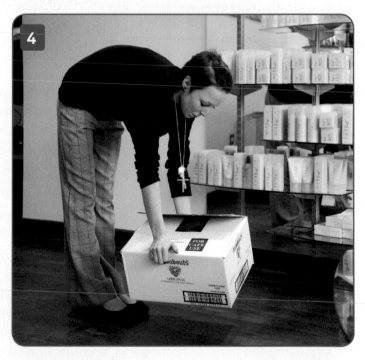

A heavy box is a hazard. It can present a high risk to someone who lifts it incorrectly, rather than someone who uses the correct manual handling techniques.

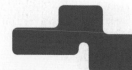

Identifying the hazards and evaluating the risks in your workplace (2)

'Get smart, get trained and get it right, first time, every time'

The Health and Safety at Work Act 1974, (see page 14 for more information) covers everyone in the salon – employees, self-employed people and visitors, such as technical reps and clients. You must be trained before you carry out any job within the salon, no matter how small or quick the task is. Failing to comply with correct working practices within the salon could harm you or your colleagues. Professional hairdressers are legally bound to abide by manufacturers' instructions, the salon policy and local bylaws.

Failure to follow the act can result in heavy penalties. Criminal proceedings, heavy fines and/or imprisonment do happen, not just to salon owners but also to the individual responsible for failing to comply. If you have any issues about health and safety, discuss them with a member of staff. Make sure the discussion is recorded, and any action required is followed up. In this unit you will learn about a variety of policies and regulations you must follow during your working life.

>> Get up and go!

Correctly name the people responsible for health and safety in your workplace. Create a flow chart detailing their name and position within the salon along with their responsibilities, e.g. Salon Manager Emma is responsible for risk assessment. Identify the person who is responsible for reporting any accidents to the Health and Safety Executive. Present this to your assessor when you have completed it.

Get ahead

Design a pack of playing cards to be used in the salon as a memory jogger and revision tool. Perhaps you could code the cards using the symbols hearts, spades, clubs and diamonds. For example, use diamonds as 'doing' cards, hearts as 'thinking' cards, clubs as 'discussion' cards and spades as 'dig and research' cards. Here are some ideas for the different kinds of activities.

- Diamonds: demonstrate how you would lift a product from a high shelf.
- Hearts: thinking about the psychology of colour and how different colours affect mood, why do salons choose the colours they do for their interiors, uniforms, etc.?
- Clubs: discuss which fire-fighting equipment can be used on electrical and non-electrical fires.
- Spades: find out what is meant by an infectious condition of the body, and why potentially infectious conditions should be reported.

Sharpen up!

Neil had been working in the salon for three months. The salon owner was keen to advance Neil's knowledge and often demonstrated hairdressing techniques to him. This included removing colours, shampooing and rinsing perms. Neil was responsible for the usual day-to-day duties, such as client care and general salon organisation.

One evening near Christmas, Neil had a lot of clients to deal with. He was asked to place a plastic cap over a client's bleached hair and place her under a dryer. Neil had been keen to learn the correct way to apply and process bleach and always read the manufacturer's instructions. He discovered dry heat was not recommended for this type of bleach and quietly explained this to the stylist. At this time the client started to complain she was uncomfortable under the hood dryer. Neil went to investigate and discovered the bleach had run down the client's neck and back, bleaching her clothes and burning her skin. Neil was then instructed to rinse the client's hair and deal with her clothes as best as he could. The client was angry that no apology was offered by the salon owner and claimed she would sue.

Who was negligent? Can the client sue both Neil and the salon owner? Discuss this situation with your colleagues.

➤➤ Get up and go!

Draw a simple plan of the hairdressing salon where you work. Walk round the salon and identify where the following are located: fire exits, specified assembly points, fire extinguishers and first aid equipment. Use a key to help explain your sketch.

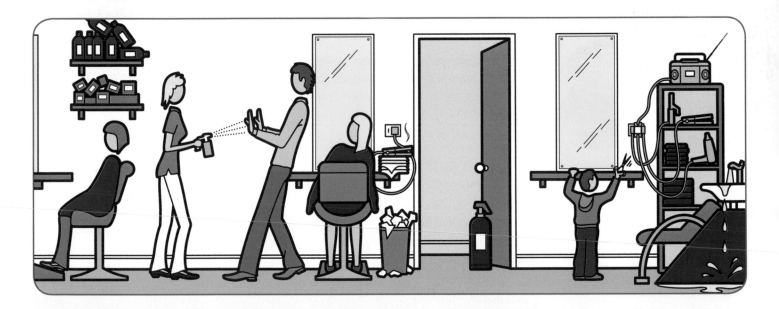

Identify the hazards in the salon above and make a list of them. Give the same exercise to another member of staff and compare your results.

Identifying the hazards and evaluating the risks in your workplace (3)

» Get up and go!

Check which of the potentially harmful working practices and aspects of your workplace presents the highest risk to you and to others. How do you control those risks within the limits of your own authority? For example, look at the pictures of slippery surfaces. What scope do you have for controlling this risk?

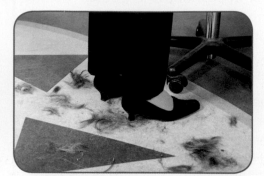
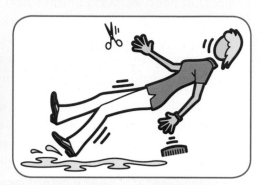

Slippery surfaces present a risk to you and your clients and can be caused by water and hair on the floor

Wearing long, loose clothes in the salon is a hazard. It may only be a low risk if the work area is clean, tidy and quiet. However, when you are expected to move quickly from one area to another, it presents a high risk as your clothing could get caught on the worktops, door handles, or perhaps on the heel of your shoe as you climb a flight of stairs.

If you find faulty equipment, pass on suggestions for reducing risks, report it to a senior colleague and make a note of the discussion.

Look at the table below and describe your responsibilities for health and safety in the salon as an employee. Discuss the completed table with a colleague. Part of the table has been completed for you.

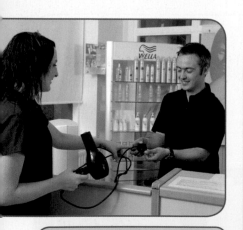

Verbally and non-verbally report any hazard to a senior member of staff, and provide evidence you have dealt with hazards which present a risk

Hazard	Risk?	Sort it?	Report it?	Control measures
Trailing flexes	Yes	Yes	Yes	Run the flex alongside the wall
Broken bulb				Check all electrics daily
Loose hair on the floor		Yes		
Broken edge on worktop				Make good until permanently repaired
Spillage on the floor			Yes	
Perm lotion running into your client's eyes	Yes			
Saturated cotton wool around the hairline			Yes	
Colour stain around the hairline				
Broken vent on hairdryer				

Within the salon you must identify working practices which could harm you or other people. Remaining alert to potential hazards will help protect everyone in the salon at any time. Remember: you need to concentrate and keep alert when dealing with products, tools and equipment.

Your physical wellbeing is essential not only to you but also to others within the salon. Too many late nights, over indulgence in food or alcohol or additional stress with personal issues will have a bearing on how you carry out your day-to-day duties. You are part of a team – if one person does not give 100% it will have a serious impact on the health and safety of the team and your clients. Make sure your behaviour does not put the health and safety of you or others in your salon at risk.

» Get up and go!

After reading the left-hand paragraphs, make a list of the potentially harmful working practices you come into contact with on a daily basis.

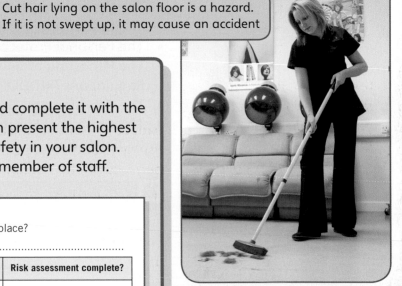

Cut hair lying on the salon floor is a hazard. If it is not swept up, it may cause an accident

» Get up and go!

Have a look at the following documentation and complete it with the help of a colleague. Report those hazards which present the highest risks to the people responsible for health and safety in your salon. When complete, check the details with a senior member of staff.

HAZARD CHECKLIST
Which hazards are present in my workplace?

Date .... Checked by ....

	Relevant to my workplace?	Risk assessment complete?
Fire		
Electric shock		
Posture		
Workplace environmental conditions		
Use of mains gas appliances		
Use and storage of chemical substances		
Hazardous substances		
Slips and trips		
Falls		
Falling objects		
Stress		
Work equipment		
Maintenance		
Infection control		
Other (list)		

? Memory jogger

Explain what the following terms mean: 'hazard'; 'risk'; 'control'.

What does the word 'alert' mean?

How does stress present itself as a hazard?

What may happen if there was a trailing wire across the salon floor?

What can you do to reduce the risk on a slippery floor?

Health and safety laws (1)

We are now going to look at the key factors within each of the health and safety laws which affect your day-to-day work. You are working with many different aspects of health and safety every day and in many cases this can be a natural process. The laws which relate to you and others in the workplace are there to protect everyone, whether they are a member of staff or a visitor to the salon. The acts you should be aware of are listed below.

- The Health and Safety at Work Act 1974
- The Fire Precautions Act 1971
- The Electricity at Work Regulations 1989
- The Workplace (Health, Safety and Welfare) Regulations 1992
- The Manual Handling Operations Regulations 1992
- The Personal Protective Equipment (PPE) at Work Regulations 1992
- The Reporting of Injuries, Diseases and Dangerous Occurrences Regulations (RIDDOR) 1995
- The Provision and Use of Work Equipment Regulations (PUWER) 1998
- The Control of Substances Hazardous to Health Regulations (COSHH) 2002

>> **Get up and go!**

Think about your responsibilities in your job. Read the list of workplace regulations above and write a simple statement about how each affects your day-to-day work in the salon. Use the diagram on page 20 to help you. This information may then be presented as part of your communications key skills short talk.

The Health and Safety at Work Act 1974

The Health and Safety at Work Act 1974 covers everyone: employees, self-employed people and visitors, such as technical reps and clients. The act covers a variety of working practices and is linked to many associated pieces of legislation covering any specific job role within any industry. The act informs both employer and employee with respect to many aspects of health and safety within the workplace and outlines everybody's duties and responsibilities.

Employers have slightly different obligations from employees. Employers are bound by a duty of care to each of their employees. This means everything an employer does when setting up and running a business will be done with the safety of all who come into contact with the business in mind. In order for this to be effective, the following must be adhered to by all employers.

- A workplace and systems of work must be provided and maintained.
- The use, handling, storage and transport of articles and substances must be accounted for.
- Information, instruction, training and supervision must be provided.
- Access and exits must be clear and free from hazard.
- The working environment, facilities and welfare arrangements must comply with the act.

The act's key message

It is your duty to maintain the health and safety of yourself and others who may be affected by your actions.

The Fire Precautions Act 1971

If you discover a fire you must raise the alarm calmly and safely. Staff, clients and visitors must be notified and escorted from the building using the nearest fire exit. Dial 999 and ask the operator for the fire service. Give the operator your name and the address of the salon, as well as brief details of the situation.

If you have been trained in fire fighting (and if the fire is small) use the most appropriate fire extinguisher to tackle the fire, but only if it is safe for you to do so.

Under the Fire Precautions Act 1971 all premises are required to have fire-fighting equipment, which must be maintained in good working order.

? Memory jogger

Who is the person responsible for reporting health and safety matters in the salon?

How would you deal with the following?

- Slippery surfaces.
- Spillages.
- Obstructions to doorways.
- Hydrogen peroxide spillage on the floor.

⟩⟩ Get up and go!

Evidence is important when creating your portfolio and within your own work role. Provide some examples of how you have taken steps to reduce health and safety risks in the salon. Take photographs and use them as evidence. Think about before and after shots.

Fire is dangerous. If you discover a fire you should treat it with caution. Breathing in hot air from a fire can damage your airways and lungs. Burning chemicals can give off toxic fumes; if you breathe in these fumes they can cause asphyxiation. Smoke-filled buildings are a health hazard because you cannot see or breathe.

Fire can damage the salon by causing decorations to smoulder, ceilings to collapse, fixtures and fittings to burn and damage to walls. Fire damage to the salon can lead to blocked passageways, which could cause a lethal hazard – someone could suffocate due to a lack of oxygen.

Health and safety laws (2)

Fire prevention and fire-fighting equipment

To put out a fire you need to be trained in dealing with a variety of different fires. You can be trained to use a fire extinguisher in order to put out small fires. To extinguish a fire you need to remove one of its three components – oxygen, heat or fuel.

> **» Get up and go!**
>
> - Find out where your fire-fighting equipment is in the salon and how often you have a fire drill.
> - What types of fire extinguisher do you have? Take photographs of each type of fire extinguisher and explain the difference to your assessor.

Types of fire extinguisher

There are many ways in which to put fires out safely and we must remember the fire extinguishers provided in the salon are there for a professional purpose. All fire extinguishers are colour coded to indicate the type of fire it can be used for.

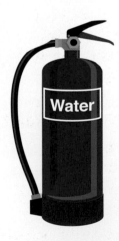 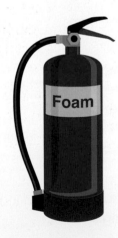 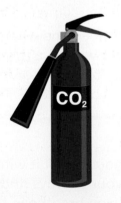 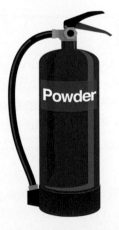 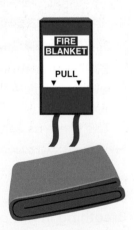

Class A A water extinguisher can be used to put out fires involving paper, coal, textiles and wood

Class B A foam extinguisher can be used to put out fires involving flammable liquids such as grease, oil, petrol and paints (but not cooking oil or grease)

Class C A carbon dioxide extinguisher can be used to put out fires involving flammable gases

Class Electrical A dry powder extinguisher can be used to put out electrical fires

Class F A blanket can be used to put out fires involving cooking oils and fats

✂ Sharpen up!

Knowing which types of extinguisher should *never* be used on which types of fire is as important as knowing which types of extinguisher *should* be used on which types of fire!

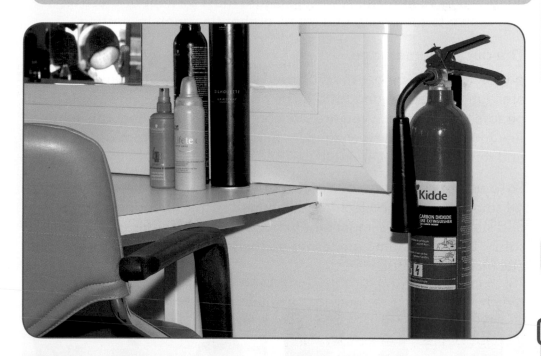

» Get up and go!

- Which types of extinguisher can be used on more than one type of fire?
- Which types of extinguisher should never be used on which types of fire?

Fire extinguishers should be easily accessible

» Get up and go!

Discuss the value of inviting a member of the Fire Brigade into your salon and asking them to talk about the different types of fire extinguisher available to you and your colleagues. Use the evidence they bring for your Health and Safety project. They may offer to give a small controlled demonstration of how to use a fire extinguisher.

Many fires could be avoided if simple house-keeping rules were applied in the workplace.

- Fire doors must be kept closed and unlocked to prevent a fire from spreading and to enable staff and visitors to leave the buildings safely.
- Keep fire exits free from rubbish at all times.
- All electrical equipment must be used in accordance with manufacturers' instructions and must be regularly inspected by a qualified electrician. Correct fuses must be fitted and sockets must not be overloaded.
- Keep aerosols away from any heat source, including the sun and radiators.
- Carelessness causes fires – look out for your own and others' safety.

? Memory jogger

What would you do if you found that a fire extinguisher in your salon was damaged?

What three things are required for a fire to start?

What is the most appropriate fire extinguisher for dealing with an electrical fire?

What could be the possible consequences of using incorrect fire equipment?

List three precautions you could take to eliminate the possibility of fire.

Health and safety laws (3)

The Electricity at Work Regulations 1989

A qualified electrician must test every electrical appliance in the salon once a year. This includes 'domestic' equipment, such as the washing machine, the fridge, the cooker and the kettle, as well as all hairdressing equipment. A written record must be kept of these tests and shown to the health and safety authorities upon inspection.

The act's key message

All electrical equipment must be used appropriately and with precaution, checked and tested. The position of plugs and sockets must be safe and the space you are working in must have adequate lighting. Any faulty or damaged equipment must be removed from use, labelled and reported to a responsible person.

Safe use and storage of electrical equipment

All salons depend on electrical equipment such as handheld hairdryers and steamers, so it is important to handle and store this equipment safely. Below are some guidelines on the safe use and storage of electrical equipment.

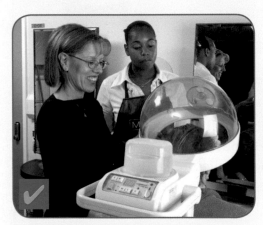

Know how to use the equipment

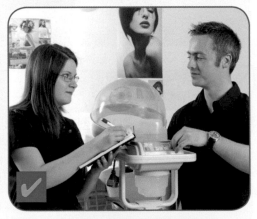

Be trained in the equipment's use

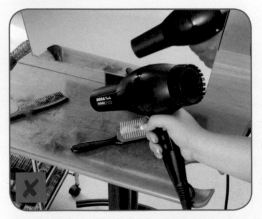

Use the equipment only for the purpose intended

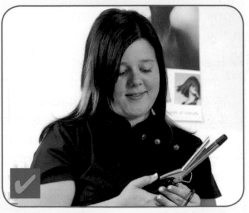

Visually check the equipment prior to use

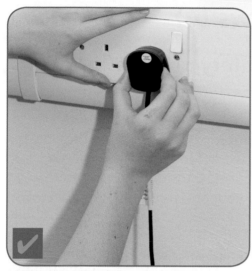

Switch off the equipment and remove from the power supply when finished

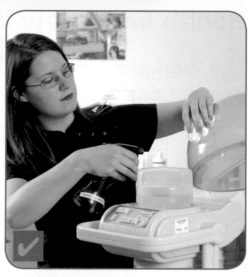

Be trained in the equipment's use

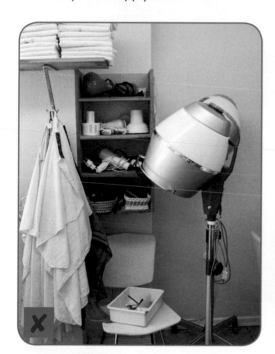

Store the equipment safely, in an allocated area

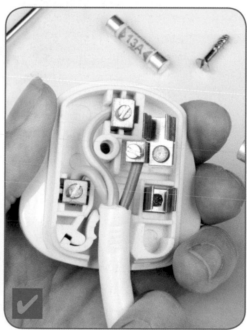

Test the equipment regularly – this should be carried out by a qualified electrician

? Memory jogger

What responsibilities do you have under the Electricity at Work Regulations?

How often should equipment be checked for damage?

Describe how you would deal with the following:

- no power to an appliance
- knotted electrical cables
- cable trapped under a heavy styling unit
- having wet hands when working with clippers
- wet salon floor
- faulty electrical equipment.

>> Get up and go!

Look at each piece of electrical equipment in your salon and find out when they were recently PAT tested. (This means a qualified electrician tests your hairdryers, clippers, tongs, etc. every twelve months, labels it with a 'Portable Appliance Test' or PAT sticker, and dates it when the test was completed.) Bring this information to your assessor and discuss your findings.

Health and safety laws (4)

The Workplace (Health, Safety and Welfare) Regulations 1992

This regulation requires all at work to help maintain a safe and healthy working environment. Every employer is required to provide a safe working environment for all at work. Make sure you follow environmentally friendly working practices. Consider the risks to the environment which may be present in your salon and in your own job.

The act's key message

When working in the salon you must maintain a safe and healthy environment.

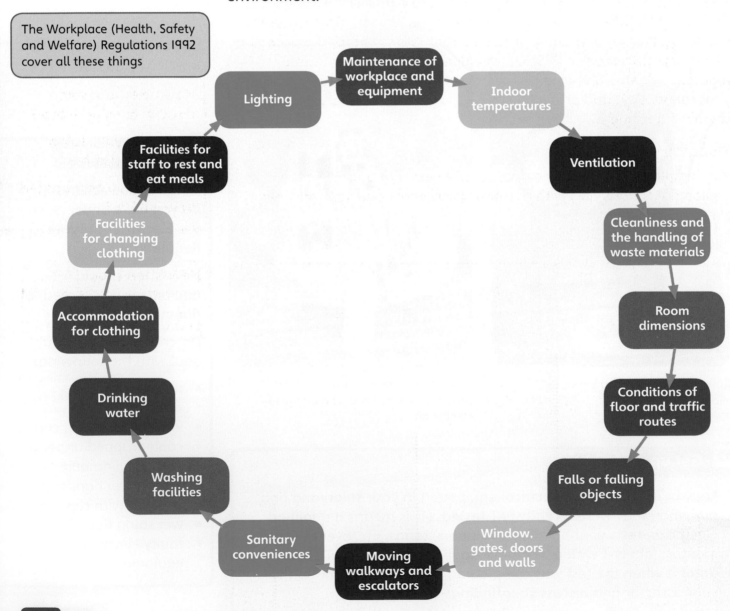

The Workplace (Health, Safety and Welfare) Regulations 1992 cover all these things

- Lighting
- Maintenance of workplace and equipment
- Indoor temperatures
- Ventilation
- Cleanliness and the handling of waste materials
- Room dimensions
- Conditions of floor and traffic routes
- Falls or falling objects
- Window, gates, doors and walls
- Moving walkways and escalators
- Sanitary conveniences
- Washing facilities
- Drinking water
- Accommodation for clothing
- Facilities for changing clothing
- Facilities for staff to rest and eat meals

» **Get up and go!**

Write a simple list of the health and safety practices you come across at work. Discuss your findings with your colleagues. You may find that some tasks are performed differently in some salons. Ask your colleagues the reasons why they have chosen to work this way and what the benefits are for them and their clients. Do they vary their working practices according to the client they are working on?

The Personal Protective Equipment (PPE) at Work Regulations 1992

These regulations state you must wear suitable protective gloves and an apron when dealing with any chemical or harmful substance. Clients must also be suitably protected during any chemical treatments. By making sure you use PPE you will meet the health and safety regulations and workplace policies. Remember, PPE includes preparing your clients' hair and protecting their skin where necessary prior to any chemical treatment.

The act's key message

Your employer must provide appropriate personal protective equipment for working with chemical treatments and you must always use it when applicable.

 Memory jogger

How does your salon dispose of salon waste?

How does your salon dispose of sharps?

Why are you encouraged to wear PPE?

Personal protective equipment must be worn when carrying out chemical treatments

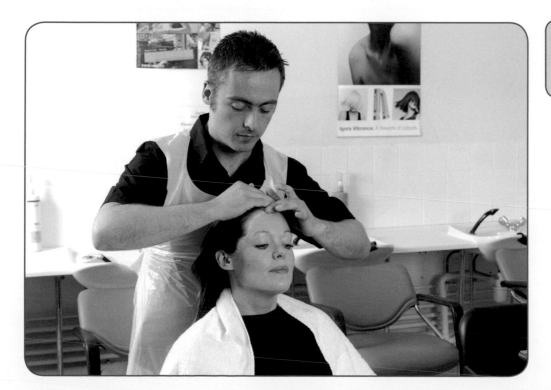

Health and safety laws (5)

The Manual Handling Operations Regulations 1992

This act requires measures such as following a set procedure when dealing with heavy or awkwardly shaped objects. The act deals with lifting items, pushing or pulling hairdressing trolleys, carrying loads and stacking shelves. All people at work must minimise the risks from lifting and handling objects.

The act's key message

This act provides guidelines for protecting yourself and others and minimising risks when lifting heavy objects.

Safe handling practices when dealing with hazards and risks

A box of heavy stock is an example of a hazard – it presents a risk to someone who needs to lift it manually, so safe handling practices must be used. The most common types of injury from lifting incorrectly are back strain and pulled muscles.

Assess the risk

Assess the box before you attempt to move it. Is it too heavy or bulky to move safely? If so, you could take out some of the items in the box before lifting or ask another member of staff for help.

If something is too heavy for you to lift on your own, ask a colleague for help

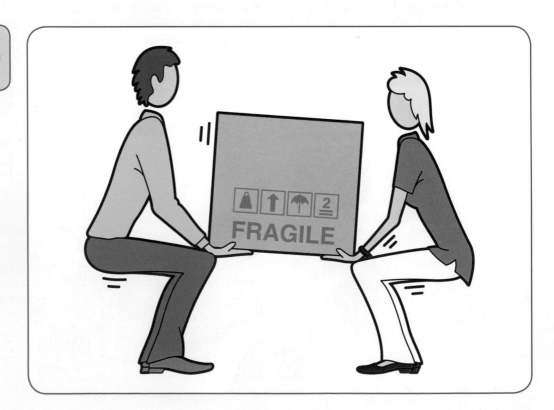

You must be trained in correct lifting practice, as with all aspects of your day-to-day work. Plan your route and remove any obstructions. Do you have a safe passageway to carry this load? Where are you going to put it down? Think about the lift you are going to carry out. Is the load to be lifted of a regular shape? Does it have sharp edges? Do you need to wear protective gloves? Are you wearing suitable clothes which will allow you to bend and move freely?

Safe lifting practices

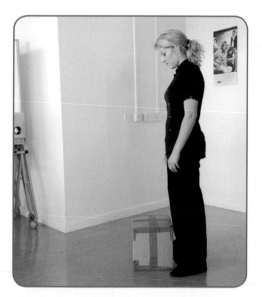

Think about the lift. Where is the load to be placed? Do you need help? Are handling aids available?

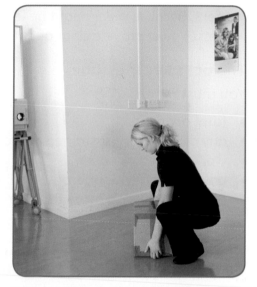

With your feet close to the load, bend your knees and keep your back straight. Tuck in your chin. Lean slightly forward over the load to get a good grip

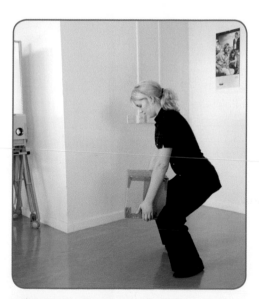

When you are sure of your grip on the load, straighten your legs and lift smoothly. Remember to keep your back straight

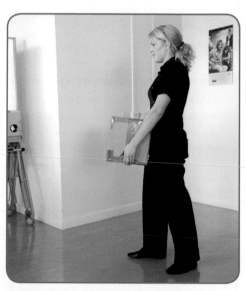

Carry the load close to your body

» Get up and go!

Watch someone the next time they lift an object from the floor. Do they bend from the hips or do they bend from the knees? How should they bend? Now practise your lifting technique using an empty box. Think about the various steps you take your own body through. Practise safe lifting practices with a colleague and then try it again on your own.

? Memory jogger

Why is it important to use the correct lifting technique?

Briefly describe how to safely lift a box of products from reception to the dispensing area.

If you had to lift a heavy box, what strategies would you consider?

Describe how to lift an item of stock from a high shelf.

Health and safety laws (6)

The Reporting of Injuries, Diseases and Dangerous Occurrences Regulations (RIDDOR) 1995

All injuries must be reported to the member of staff responsible for health and safety. The salon accident book must be completed with basic personal details of the person (or people) involved and a detailed description of the incident. Because there might be legal consequences due to the injury, all witnesses must provide clear and accurate details of what happened.

The act's key message

You must report:

- fatal accidents
- any major injury sustained at work
- work-related diseases
- any potentially dangerous event which takes place at work
- accidents causing more than three days' absence from work.

A page from an accident book

ACCIDENT REPORT FORM

SECTION 1 PERSONAL DETAILS

Full name of first aider/staff member _____

Position held in salon: _____

Date: _____

Accident (injury) ☐   Incident (illness) ☐

Time and date of accident/incident: _____

Full name of injured/ill person: _____

Staff member ☐   Client ☐   Other ☐

Address: _____

Tel. no: _____

SECTION 2 ACCIDENT/INCIDENT DETAILS

Describe what happened. In the case of an accident, state clearly what the injured person was doing. _____
_____

Name and address/tel. no. of witness(es), if any: _____
_____

Action taken

Ambulance called ☐   Taken to hospital ☐   Sent to hospital ☐   First aid given ☐

Taken home ☐   Sent home ☐   Returned to work ☐

SECTION 3 PREVENTATIVE ACTION

Preventative action implemented ☐

Describe action taken: _____
_____

Date implemented: _____

Signature of first aider/staff member: _____

Signature salon manager/owner: _____

Date: _____

Locate your salon's accident book. Look at the information contained within the book.

- Does it break the Data Protection Act?
- Can you identify the person/people who have had an accident in the salon?
- How available and visible should the accident book be?
- Where should it be stored?
- Where are the personal details related to those persons who have had an accident kept?

Discuss your findings with a colleague and then with your assessor.

The Provision and Use of Work Equipment Regulations (PUWER) 1998

These regulations lay down important health and safety controls on the provision and use of work equipment. Employers must provide equipment for use which is properly constructed, suitable for its purpose and kept in good working order. Training on how to use each piece of equipment must be provided by the employer. Staff who use the salon equipment must be competent in its use.

The act's key message

You must be competent when using tools and equipment in the salon.

Walk around your salon and look at some of the tools and equipment. If it is helpful, take a photo of each piece of equipment. Look at the equipment objectively and make a note of the state of repair of each piece.

- Is it in good working order?
- Does it need to be thrown away?
- Can it be repaired?

Let your assessor know your conclusions.

Health and safety laws (7)

The Control of Substances Hazardous to Health (COSHH) Regulations 2002

Chemicals, including perm lotions, neutralisers and hydrogen peroxide, are hazardous and present a high risk. They must be handled, stored, used and disposed of correctly in accordance with COSHH 2002. This means every chemical and product used within the salon must be assessed for risk.

Find out about the working practices within your salon and those which are relevant to your job description. It's easy to forget the risks involved in using shampoos and conditioners – remember, the ingredients can sometimes cause skin and scalp irritation. All manufacturers are duty-bound to inform you of the ingredients in each hairdressing product stored in your salon. Each item must be catalogued in a register for staff to access so all staff who are trained can deal with the possible dangers of the products they use.

Many products, such as hairspray, mousse, perm lotion and hydrogen peroxide, are potentially hazardous and should be stored in a cool, dark, locked fire-proof cabinet, preferably on a low shelf.

Potentially hazardous products should be stored correctly

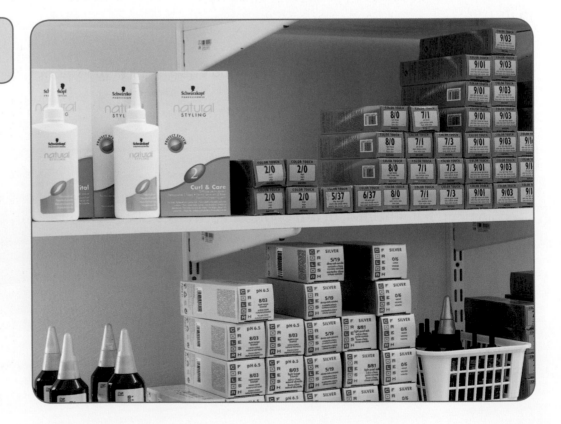

Always read and follow salon instructions, suppliers' or manufacturers' instructions and follow legal requirements as appropriate. This is very important when working with products, equipment and materials. Should you find a difference between salon, suppliers' or manufacturers' instructions you must report this to a senior member of staff. This will help you make the correct decision when using products and equipment on your clients. You must use products for their intended professional purpose only.

An example of a manufacturer's product instructions

Sharpen up!

Remember: good ventilation is important when mixing colours and bleaches and when using colouring preparations. Windows and/or an air vent must be opened, as chemicals can be dangerous if inhaled.

HYDROGEN PEROXIDE SOLUTION

Composition
Stabilised acidic aqueous solutions or emulsions containing hydrogen peroxide of various strengths for use with:

Permanent Colorants
Bleach powder
Permanent waves as neutralisers

Ingredients
Hydrogen peroxide
Hair tighteners Colorant remover up to 40 vol or 12%
Preparations containing higher concentrations of hydrogen peroxide are outside the scope of the Cosmetics Directive. In such cases, seek the advice of the supplier regarding COSHH assessments.

Hazards identification
Irritant to eyes and skin.

First-aid measures
Eyes: Rinse eyes immediately with plenty of water. If irritation persists seek medical advice.
Skin: Wash skin immediately with water. If irritation persists seek medical advice.
Ingestion: Seek medical advice immediately.

Accidental release measures
Always use water to dilute and mop up spillages.

Handling and storage
Always use non-metallic utensils to avoid rapid decomposition of the product. Do not allow contact with easily combustible materials such as paper. Store in cool, dry place away from sunlight and other sources of heat. Always store hydrogen peroxide in the container supplied. It is particularly important that no contamination enters the containers as this could lead to decomposition resulting in the liberation of heat and oxygen. Therefore, replace cap immediately after use.

Exposure controls/personal protection
Always wear suitable protective gloves. Avoid contact with eyes and face. Do not use on abraded or sensitive skin.

Stability and reactivity
Hydrogen peroxide may react with other chemicals to form dangerous materials (e.g. explosive). Therefore, avoid mixtures other than recognised formulations. Combustion may occur if hydrogen peroxide is allowed to dry out on materials such as paper, hair, wood, etc.

Disposal
Wash down the drain with plenty of water. Do not incinerate.

Memory jogger

Why should infectious conditions be reported to your salon manager?

Give an example of what might be an infectious condition.

What does COSHH stand for?

For what reason do you store harmful substances in a locked cupboard?

Why do salons have accident books?

What would you do next if you accidently cut a client's ear?

Briefly describe your duties for health and safety relating to the following regulations:

- RIDDOR
- PUWER
- COSHH

The act's key message

Any substances used in your salon could be hazardous to health and should be stored, handled, used and disposed of according to legislation, manufacturers' instructions and local bylaws.

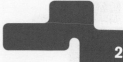

Workplace policies (I)

» Get up and go!

Find out if the salon where you work has a workplace policy.

- Do you have a member of staff who is qualified in first aid?
- How would you contact the first aider?
- What happens in the salon when the first aider is absent?

If there are more than five people employed in your salon, a workplace policy is required. The policy is written to clarify what the risks are at work on a day-to-day basis, to bring to your attention any precautions which may be necessary and to clarify who is responsible.

All members of staff must cooperate with the workplace policy to make sure the salon is a safe and healthy place to work. This should include checking that work areas are kept clean, fire exits are not blocked and you have enough space to work comfortably without bumping into work stations or other salon staff.

» Get up and go!

Complete the missing word(s) from each of the following health and safety laws:

- Fire P_____ Act (1971)
- Health and S_____ Act (1974)
- Electricity at W_____ Regulations (1989)
- Workplace _____Regulations (1992)
- Manual H_____ Operations Regulations (1992)
- Personal Protective E_____ at Work Regulations (1992)
- Reporting of Injuries, D_____, and Dangerous Occurrences Regulations (1995)
- Provision and U____ of Work Equipment Regulations (1998)
- Control of S_____ Hazardous to Health Regulations (2002)

Sterilising equipment

Sterilising equipment will ensure a hygienic working environment, preventing the risk of cross-infection and infestation. It also promotes a high standard of cleanliness to your clients. Equipment must be cleaned thoroughly before using any sterilising method. The methods of sterilisation available in the salon may include:

- barbicide
- ultraviolet
- autoclave.

You must use tools and equipment which are clean, safe and fit for their purpose – tools and equipment identified at the time of consultation must be readily available to use for professional purposes. This might include pintail combs to weave sections of hair, highlighting hooks to pull strands of hair through a highlighting cap, or professional foil strips to assist colouring. Equipment should be cleaned and sterilised as soon as possible after use to ensure it is ready for the next treatment.

Barbicide

The most popular method of sterilising is barbicide. Barbicide is quick and easy to use, but will only inhibit the growth of bacteria. You must read and follow the manufacturer's instructions when making up the solution and you must remember to change it daily.

Ultraviolet

Placing tools which are clean and dry in an ultraviolet cabinet will prevent the growth of bacteria. You must remember to turn your tools every 15 minutes to sterilise them all over.

Autoclave

The most effective method of sterilising is the autoclave, which will completely destroy all living bacteria on the surface of your tools. However, not all equipment can withstand the heat of an autoclave – temperatures reach up to 125°C!

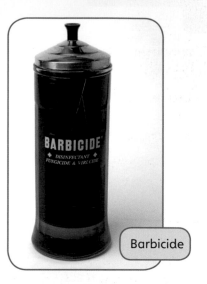

Barbicide

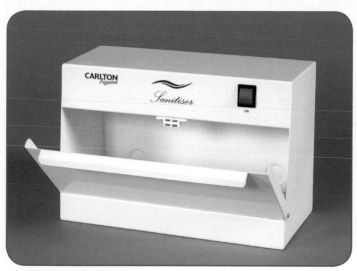

Ultraviolet cabinet

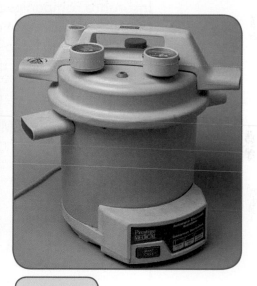

Autoclave

? **Memory jogger**

Which is the most effective method of sterilising salon equipment?

Describe the method for using an ultraviolet cabinet.

» **Get up and go!**

Are your salon's practices safe? Find out if there are any differences between your salon's workplace policies and suppliers' or manufacturers' instructions in relation to day-to-day practical jobs. Think about neutralising, rinsing off a colour and blow-drying a client's hair. These are practical activities, which are carried out every day in every salon, and you will find that practices vary.

Workplace policies (2)

Public- and treatment-liability insurance

Did you know all salons are duty-bound to take out public- and treatment-liability insurance? If a member of staff were to injure one of your clients in the salon as a result of negligence, the client would have grounds to sue the member of staff and the salon.

The employer's insurance certificate must cover all staff, clients and visitors to the salon and must be displayed for all to read, should they wish. The name of the insurance company, the salon name and address, the nature of the business and the start date and renewal date will be included. The salon will have to renew this certificate of insurance every year.

The insurance company requires evidence if a claim is made. They must be certain all reasonable steps were taken to prevent the situation occurring. Were all tests carried out correctly and recorded? Were the manufacturer's instructions read, understood and followed?

Insurance companies do not always pay out on the claims they receive if they are suspicious of negligent practices. Should this be the case, where is the money going to come from? Will the salon owner have to sell the salon? Will you have to find the money yourself if you were responsible?

An employer's liability insurance certificate

CERTIFICATE OF EMPLOYER'S LIABILITY INSURANCE (A)

(Where required by regulation 5 of the Employer's Liability (Compulsory Insurance) Regulations 1998 (the Regulations), one or more copies of this certificate must be displayed in each place of business at which the policy holder employs persons covered by the policy.)

Policy No   **R3/21LG52123**
Reference No   92L31
1. Name of policy holder   Mrs Tiffany Tsang trading as Top Tips
2. Date of commencement of insurance policy   31 July 2004
3. Date of expiry of insurance   31 July 2005

We hereby certify that subject to paragraph 2:-
1. The policy to which this certificate relates satisfies the requirements of the relevant law applicable in Great Britain, Northern Ireland, the Isle of Man, the Island of Jersey, the Island of Guernsey and the Island of Alderney (b); and
2 (a) the minimum amount of cover provided by this policy is no less than £5 million (c). Signed on behalf of EverSure plc (Authorised Insurer)
R J Stanley
CHIEF EXECUTIVE OFFICER UK

Notes
(a) Where the employer is a company to which regulation 3(2) of the Regulations applies, the certificate shall state in a prominent place, either that the policy covers the holding company and all its subsidiaries, or that the policy covers the holding company and all its subsidiaries except any specially excluded by name, or that the policy covers the holding company and only the name subsidiaries.
(b) Specify applicable law as provided for in regulation 4(5) of the Regulations.
(c) See regulation 3(1) of the Regulations and delete whichever of paragraphs 2(a) or 2(b) does not apply. Where 2(b) is applicable, specify the amount of cover provided by the relevant policy.
paragraph 2(b) does not apply and is deleted.

YOUR CERTIFICATE OF EMPLOYER'S LIABILITY INSURANCE IS ATTACHED ABOVE.
THE EMPLOYER'S LIABILITY (COMPULSORY INSURANCE) REGULATIONS 1998 REQUIRE YOU TO KEEP THIS CERTIFICATE OR A COPY FOR 40 YEARS.

Please fold as shown and insert the certificate in the protective cover provided. A copy of the certificate must be displayed at all places where you employ persons covered by the policy. Extra copies of the certificate are available on request.

Situation vacant

Specific duties related to health and safety should be stated in your job description and made clear to you at interview. Below is an example of a job description for you and your colleagues to discuss.

Job Description	Post Holder Junior
Job Title	Junior
Place of Work	Cutting Creations, Aylesbury

Candidate Specification

The successful candidate will
- Have good interpersonal skills; demonstrate a professional level of client care
- Be flexible and willing to work as a team member
- Work Saturdays and at least one late evening each week
- Take responsibility for securing models for practice and assessment purposes
- Update practical skills regularly at training sessions
- Take an active interest in all aspects of work within the salon
- Attend hairdressing seminars and professional courses in order to keep abreast of current and emerging techniques
- Demonstrate appropriate health and safety practices when working in the salon
- Complete the appropriate hairdressing qualification within the specified timeframe
- Undertake other reasonable duties as required by senior staff

Specific duties
Undertake day-to-day duties such as
- Shampoo and condition hair and scalp
- Assist with perming, relaxing, neutralising, and colouring for both European and African type hair
- Assist with salon reception duties
- Sell retail products
- Make refreshments
- Reduce the risks to general health and safety by taking reasonable care, co-operating with requests made by senior staff and not interfering with or misusing any piece of equipment, tools or products
- Sterilise equipment
- Continuous preparation for hairdressing treatments and maintain the salon work areas
- Wash and dry towels and gowns
- Stock checking

About the salon and our staff
We are a friendly team who enjoy busy professional lives. We strive for perfection, sincerity and honesty in everything we do.

Our skills are updated on a regular basis by attending regular seminars and holding regular teach-in evenings. We look forward to working with you and wish you an enjoyable and rewarding time with us.

The candidate will enjoy
- Two weeks' paid holiday each year
- The national minimum wage
- A 40-hour working week
- 9am – 6pm (1 hour for lunch every day)

Dear Dana,

I have recently seen an advertisement in the Hairdressers Journal and I am interested in applying for the job. My hair is mousy brown and I thought it could do with spicing up a bit. I know it is important to look my best when I attend interviews. I really am worried about my appearance. Can you help?

Yours sincerely,

Lisa

A job description

Dana says:

It would be a good idea to go to the salon and ask for their advice and guidance about different types of colour, but say you do not want to commit to a colour. Ask about suitable temporary products and listen to what they say. Do they have coloured hair mascara, temporary colours or perhaps semi-permanent colours? Look around the salon and decide if you would like to come back for an interview or if would rather look elsewhere.

The opportunity this experience presents will stand you in good stead when dealing with prospective employers. Remember, all job interviews are different and the experience is invaluable. By taking this approach you will have obtained some sound advice about how to colour your hair and, because you have visited the salon, you will be able to make an informed decision about your job application. If you like what the salon suggested, book an appointment and view the salon from a client's perspective.

Good luck!

Dana

? Memory jogger

Think of three safe practices when using colouring and bleaching products.

What effect could unprofessional behaviour have on your colleagues and clients?

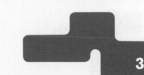

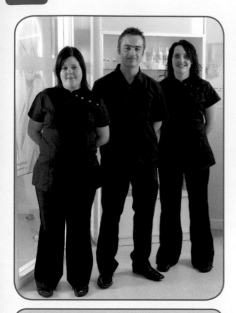

High standards of personal presentation and professional dress create a good first impression for clients

Get up and go!

Carry out a small survey of various salons in your area and find out what their staff wear. Bring your findings back to your salon and discuss them with your colleagues. For safe working practices within the salon, you need to think about the most appropriate materials to wear. Write down the most suitable types of materials your tops, skirts and trousers must be made from.

Personal presentation and behaviour (I)

First impressions are very important. People can form an opinion of you within a few seconds of meeting you. They will judge you on the way you look and the way you behave. Imagine how clients would feel if you arrived at your salon looking as if you had just fallen out of bed! Do you think they would want you to do their hair if you looked like you could not take care of your own appearance? The way you look really matters. However good your hairdressing skills may be, if you look untidy and unwashed, the image you present will give clients a bad impression.

One of the most important things to remember is the appearance of any salon must be one of cleanliness, tidiness and good organisation. Your first impression when you go into a salon will help you to make your mind up whether or not you would want to be a client or member of staff there. If the salon appears to be clean, tidy and run efficiently you are more likely to think it is a nicer place to be than somewhere dirty or untidy.

First impressions count

Many rules and regulations will form a part of your everyday life in the salon. Equally important to your day-to-day work is your personal presentation. Your personal presentation should be a total image, from head to foot, of safety and professionalism.

Dressed for success!

Clothes must be neat and streamlined, so no flowing skirts, trousers or loose baggy tops. Black tends to be the industry's preferred colour, although this varies from salon to salon. Make sure your personal presentation and behaviour in the salon:

- protects the health and safety of you and other people
- meets legal responsibilities
- complies with salon instructions.

Sometimes fashion shoes look great but are not always good for your feet. You will spend a lot of time on your feet when you are working in the salon and it is important to choose shoes which fit properly and meet certain health and safety requirements. Choose full-covered leather shoes with closed-in toes and low heels. Leather allows the feet to breathe and will help prevent unpleasant foot odour. Full-covered shoes are worn in the salon for health and safety reasons – they will protect your feet if you drop something sharp on them. Sensible shoes will also stop hairs from becoming stuck in the soles of your feet!

> **》 Get up and go!**
>
> Think of the reasons behind the following statements about salon dress.
>
> - Your clothes must be streamlined and not baggy.
> - You must always wear full-covered shoes or boots with a low heel and sole.

Personal hygiene

Hairdressers are constantly on their feet and work in close proximity to their clients and colleagues. Your clothes must be clean and pressed on a daily basis. You must shower daily and use a suitable deodorant. Tops must meet the waistband of your trousers or skirt – your client does not necessarily want to see your pierced navel or recent tattoo. Tops must also have sleeves, short or long. When you lift your arms up to work on your client's hair, they do not want to see your underarm hair or smell an unwashed armpit! Smells can linger, so try to avoid spicy meals during the week. Remember too that the smell of cigarette smoke can linger on your clothing and breath.

> **》 Get up and go!**
>
> Think about the causes of bad breath. How can you avoid these? Discuss with a colleague various ways in which to prevent bad breath.

Conversation topics to avoid

Conduct also falls within your personal presentation. All you say and do is part and parcel of you as a professional person. It is pointless being correctly dressed only to follow it through with inappropriate conversation and conduct. Topics of conversation to stay away from are personal issues such as sex, drugs, religion and politics. These topics of conversation can cause friction within the salon and are best avoided. Remember: the client is your primary concern so you must demonstrate a professional, business-like approach to all aspects of the client's visit.

Personal presentation and behaviour (2)

Efficient working practices

By positioning your tools within easy reach and keeping them well organised you will make efficient use of your time and working area. Being well prepared and organised will also present a professional image to your clients. Remove waste at the end of all perming, colouring and lightening treatments and dispose of it in line with local bylaws. This will leave your work surfaces free from any risk or hazard and will present a tidy working area.

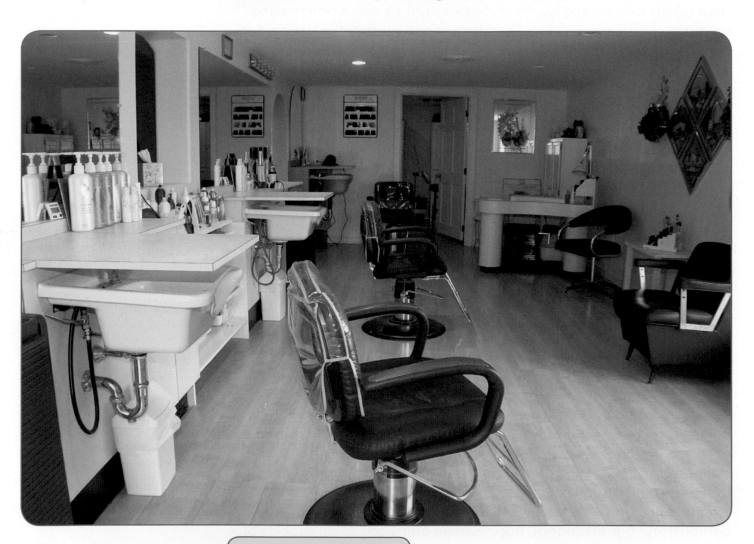

A well-organised working area will give your clients a good first impression

Personal conduct

Personal conduct covers all areas of your working life, from dealing with clients and other members of staff to eating and drinking. What kind of an impression would you create if you ate in your work area?

Are you an extrovert who likes to show everyone how happy you are? What kind of an impression does your behaviour create? Be happy and remember, good personal conduct demonstrates to your clients how professional you are. Sensible behaviour means potential accidents are prevented, you promote a healthy and safe place to work and the Health and Safety Act is respected.

General behaviour in the salon includes body language. If you do not agree with something, does it show in your body language? Consider whether taking drugs (either obtained legally by a doctor or illegally) affects your colleagues and clients, as well as your standard of work. Always remember to check out the salon's policy for smoking and alcohol.

Finally, conduct also includes reporting staff absence and punctual timekeeping. This means you must inform your employer of any absence and indicate your expected return date. This will enable your manager to reorganise your work schedule and allocate jobs to other members of staff.

≫ Get up and go!

Think about how you would hand over to a member of staff at the end of a day.

What about the appointments for tomorrow? Have they all been accounted for in terms of resources? This needs to be done on a nightly basis just like your cashing up procedures in reception.

Suggest a handover process to your line manager and trial it for a period of time, refine it and put it into place as a standard practice.

? Memory jogger

How does personal presentation affect health and safety in the salon?

List three ways you can keep your breath fresh.

How can you make sure you do not have body odour?

Your colleague has long hair. How might this affect health and safety in the salon? What can she do to minimise risk?

Describe positive body language in the salon.

Safe working practices

In this unit you have covered the many different aspects of health and safety. You have learned that to work in the hairdressing industry, you will always need to demonstrate you understand the health and safety requirements and policies in the salon. This knowledge will provide present and future employers with a professional employee who can demonstrate an approved code of practice for maintaining a safe and healthy working environment.

Health and safety at work

Health means being well, both physically and mentally. Safety means being free from risk of danger and injury. In order to stay well in everyday life, we need:

- shelter, food and drink
- clean air
- space to work and move around
- an ambient temperature
- freedom of movement with no risk of harm.

Safety and comfort for you and your client

We have looked at the reasons why everyone is required to behave safely and professionally. You must take reasonable care for the health and safety of yourself and others who may be affected by what you do. You must also cooperate with your employer, salon owner or manager to ensure health and safety procedures are followed.

Further information

Use the following sources to further develop your knowledge and understanding of this unit.

Websites

You can find useful information on the websites for the following organisations:

- Health and Safety Executive
- COSHH Essentials
- UK Fire Service
- NHS Plus

Books and leaflets

- Health and Safety Executive: priced and free publications are available from HSE Books. Tel: 01787 881165 or visit their website.

Organisations

- Contact the British Occupational Hygiene Society (BOHS) on 01332 298101 or visit their website to find out more about occupational hygiene.
- Look in the Yellow Pages under 'Health and safety consultants', 'Health authorities and services' or 'Occupational health'.

Look at the list of employment-related acts and regulations in the left-hand column of the table, most of which you have learned about in this unit. Match them with the appropriate statement in the right-hand column, for example: **N** Equal Opportunities Legislation (Amended 2003) is matched with **4** Everyone should be treated equally as an individual, regardless of their race, religion or disability.

Act or regulation	Statement
A Health and Safety at Work Act (1974)	**I** Accidents must be written in the salon accident book and serious injuries must be reported to the local enforcement officer.
B Electricity at Work Regulations (1989)	**2** Salons that hold client information on a computer must register with the Data Protection Register, and all information must be kept confidential and available to the client if they wish to see it. The salon must not threaten to or misuse information.
C Control of Substances Hazardous to Health (COSSH) Regulations (2002)	**3** Employers must provide free of charge all necessary personal protective equipment for employees.
D Personal Protective Equipment (PPE) at Work Regulations (1992)	**4** Everyone should be treated equally as an individual, regardless of their race, religion or disability.
E The Provision and Use of Work Equipment Regulations (PUWER) (1998)	**5** The salon must be kept safe and clean, and employees must obey salon rules.
F Employer's Liability Act (1998)	**6** All people at work must know how to minimise their risk of injury from lifting and handling objects.
G Fire Precautions Act (1971)	**7** This law applies to the storage, use and disposal of all hairdressing products and chemicals.
H The Cosmetic Products Regulations (2004)	**8** Hairdressing chemicals and waste must be disposed of safely.
I Environmental Protection Act (2005)	**9** This is an insurance cover for employers and employees in the event of accidents to themselves and their clients.
J Workplace Regulation (1992)	**10** This law covers the rules which recommend the different volumes and strengths of hydroxide-based products, i.e. hydrogen peroxide.
K Manual Handling Operations Regulations (2002)	**II** This act is designed to protect everyone involved in working situations. It states the responsibilities of both employers and employees regarding health and safety in the workplace.
L Reporting of Injuries, Diseases and Dangerous Occurrences Regulations (RIDDOR) (1995)	**12** All fire-fighting equipment must be in good working order, be suitable for the types of fire likely to occur and be readily available.
M Data Protection Act (2003)	**13** This law states that a qualified electrician must check every electrical appliance every 12 months.
N Equal Opportunities Legislation (Amended 2003)	**14** The employer has a duty to select equipment for use at work which is properly constructed and kept in good repair.

Note: the content of this table was correct at time of printing.

Remember – it is good practice to check regularly for amendments to keep yourself up to date.

UNIT G2

Assist with salon reception duties

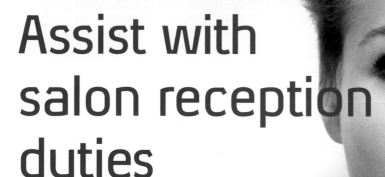

Image by TONI&GUY

First impressions count to a lot of people. Whether about you as an individual or the salon as a whole, the overall impression the client receives when they enter your place of work is very important. Within the first few seconds, your client is making a judgement about everything they see and hear. Look at your reception area. Is it clean, tidy, welcoming and professional?

This unit is about assisting with salon reception duties. You will have to demonstrate that you can keep the reception area neat and tidy, welcome people entering the salon, deal with their questions and make straightforward appointments. Using good communication skills when people come into the salon, or when they telephone the salon, is an important part of this unit.

In this unit you will learn how to:

- Maintain the reception area
- Attend to clients and enquiries
- Help to make appointments for salon services.

Here are some key words you will meet in this unit:

Communication – can be verbal (words) or non-verbal (body language, etc.)

Clients – the people who come into the salon and pay for a treatment

Enquiry – a request for information

Stationery – note paper, letter headed paper, envelopes, compliment slips, etc.

Hospitality – a gesture of giving, e.g. hot or cold drinks, magazines, looking after the client

Recording – taking a note of information, usually an appointment time and service in the appointment book

Confidentiality – respect and privacy of an individual's information

DPA – the Data Protection Act

Body language – communicating using your body, e.g. facial expressions, body movements, how you sit or stand

Retail – selling products such as shampoo and conditioner to your clients

Policy – the terms and conditions laid down by a business; course of action followed when faced with a particular situation

Maintain the reception area (I)

The reception area is the first part of the salon visitors see. You may be the first person in the salon your clients come into contact with. First impressions are important. The way in which people are dealt with will affect whether they want to come back. How you conduct yourself and treat clients can affect your salon's existing and future success.

The reception area – is it clean and tidy?

Is your salon reception area clean, tidy and welcoming? Put yourself in the place of a client and look at your reception critically. Would you feel as if you were in a professional salon? Not all salons have a separate reception area, but even so, the area in which the client is welcomed must be professionally presented. It is your duty to make sure the reception area is clean and tidy at all times.

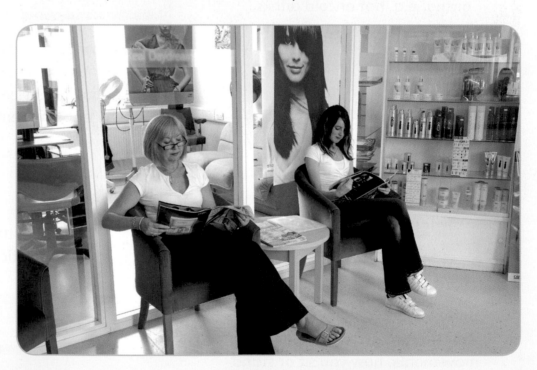

The reception area is the 'shop window' of the salon – it needs to give clients a good impression

Retail products

Your salon may sell a range of retail products. It is your job to display these neatly and to make sure the display is kept fully stocked, clean, dust-free and tidy at all times. This will encourage clients to look at the products and will also help them to decide whether they want to pick one up and buy it. This type of work is best done when the salon is quiet. It may be first thing in the morning or there may be quiet times during the day when you could dust and rearrange the products on display.

Remember, all staff must be fully aware of products stocked by the salon and how to use them. When discussing the benefits of the products with clients, you must only state what the product itself says. If you give misleading or incorrect information you may have to deal with an angry client, which could be difficult. The knowledge and understanding you learn from your technical reps will prove invaluable when you discuss products with your clients.

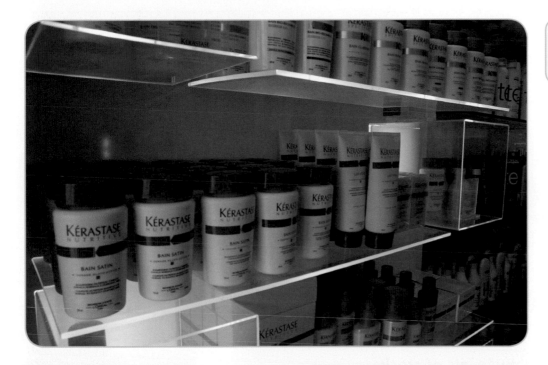

Retail product displays should look good so clients are tempted to buy!

≫ Get up and go!

Make suitable suggestions to your assessor about how you would like to display products and stock in the reception area of your salon. Where products are on display, think about using empty boxes or bottles. This will help to prevent theft. If stock losses can be kept to a minimum, this will directly affect your salon's final profit. Make a simple list of the most popular salon retail products and list the cost of each product. You may find this information useful when dealing with enquiries.

Sharpen up!

Who should you report low levels of stationery and products to in your salon? Did you know women spend more on retail products than men?

Maintain the reception area (2)

Security of stock

It is vital to keep the salon's stock secure. Small items can be removed easily without anyone noticing. The thief may be a visitor to the salon or even a member of staff. Stock should be regularly checked against actual sales to show whether anything is missing.

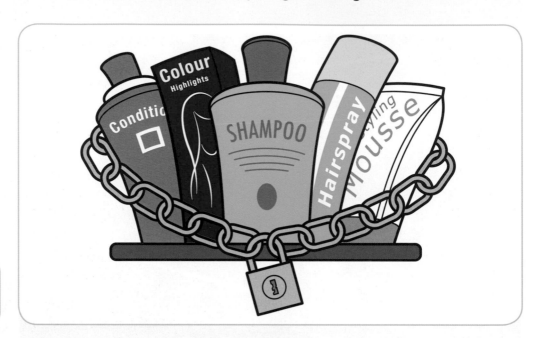

Make it difficult for thieves to take your salon's stock

Low levels of stock

As well as hair styling and treatment products and equipment, you will need a variety of other resources to help you do your job, such as stationery. Take a regular stock check of pencils, erasers, pencil sharpeners, rulers, appointment pages/books, calculators and message pads, as well as salon products. You will also need to regularly check you have enough change in the till. Promptly reporting stock shortages can make the difference between offering a professional service and making an appointment, closing a sale, or irritating the client by making him or her wait.

WELLA HAIR PRODUCTS	
Wella Lifetex Shampoo	£4.50
Wella Lifetex Mousse Conditioners	£4.80
Wella Lifetex Intensive Conditioners	£4.60
Wella High Hair Product Samples	£1.99 each or
	3 for £5.00
Wella Hair Mascara	£3.50

A retail products list

Faulty products

Sometimes accidents happen and stock may become damaged. Remove all faulty products from the reception area as soon as you can and report them to the person who controls the stock. Look for faulty stock as you prepare it for sale, for example, damaged or loose packaging, cracks or splits in bottles, leaks, and so on. Removing faulty products is essential to the smooth running of the reception area and can mean the difference between a client buying a product or not.

Many salons operate commission on all retail products sold, so it pays to be alert when dealing with stock.

Looking after your clients

Clients like to be looked after. Be friendly and polite, and remember to offer them a drink and something to read. Make sure the newspapers and magazines you offer are suitable for a general age range and are up to date. Your salon may have a client care policy of offering both non-alcoholic and alcoholic drinks. This is sometimes free to the client as part of the salon's hospitality.

It is good practice to offer refreshments when clients are waiting for the stylist to attend to them. It gives the client a feeling that something is happening.

Some salons have a video playing showing the different types of work the salon offers. This can reassure the client as they see the level of care and professionalism taken to produce the video.

▶▶ Get up and go!

Find out where the following items are kept in your salon:

- Cups and saucers.
- Glasses.
- Plastic cups for children.
- Soft drinks for children.

Where do you get more stock of coffee, tea, sugar and milk?

? Memory jogger

What does the word 'professional' mean to you?

What are the advantages of selling retail products (see the list on page 42)?

How does your salon keep its stock secure?

Who do you report low stock levels to?

What incentive would you offer staff for selling retail products?

What is the total cost, without using a calculator, for two shampoos and three intensive conditioners?

Attend to clients and enquiries (I)

Imagine you have walked into your salon for the first time and you want to find out how much a haircut is. How would it feel to be a client? The salon reception area is often a busy place, and it needs to look inviting, so when carrying out reception duties you will need to maintain a professional area of work and behave professionally at all times.

Welcoming people is what your job is all about. Make them feel special and let them know you are pleased to see them. Be knowledgeable about your area of work and speak with confidence and pride about the services your salon offers. You will need to discuss the range of treatments and their timings with a range of clients and will therefore need to learn about them.

Always stay calm and in control of any situation which arises and, if necessary, contact a senior member of staff if you find the situation becomes too difficult to deal with.

Personal appearance

When working in the reception area, your personal appearance is paramount to the success of attracting and maintaining clients. Your clothing should be neat, clean and professional at all times. Choose a suitable hairstyle to reflect your salon's standards. If you are male, are you clean shaven or growing a beard? First thing in the morning you need to shave if you are usually clean shaven. If you wear a beard, then keep it clean and well trimmed. Some make-up may help to give you a professional look and simple jewellery is better for working during the day. How about your shoes? Will they support your feet during the day without too much discomfort? Adopting these simple practices will help to give your clients confidence, paving the way to an enjoyable salon visit.

A positive and polite manner

Communication is a vital part of reception work. It is important to the success of the business. Your salon will probably have a precise greeting they will want you to use such as 'Good morning/afternoon. My name is Adrienne. May I help you?' Get into the habit of using standard professional statements and they will become second nature to you.

Smile when dealing with people who are making enquiries, be attentive and help them in a positive and polite manner. This will help the person to decide if he or she wants to return to your salon. Always show positive body language – clients may pick up on negative body language and decide to leave and not return.

There are two types of communication:

- Verbal communication uses the spoken word, either face to face or over the telephone.
- Non-verbal communication, for example, is when you write down a message or an appointment for a client. It can also mean reading, listening, or the body language you use such as nodding, smiling, frowning, and sign language. Written messages must be clear. It is often a good idea to take the message to the person concerned for his or her immediate attention.

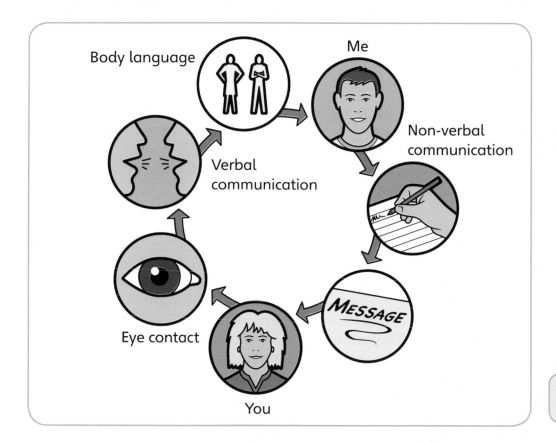

Verbal and non-verbal communication

Communication needs to be effective and clear to everyone involved. Speak at a suitable pace and use everyday business-like language, i.e. avoid using technical jargon or slang. Use an interesting and pleasant tone of voice and use appropriate open and closed questions for the client you are attending to. When a client makes an appointment, you will need to repeat the information back to him or her to make sure both you and the client understand it. Smile, look attentive and interested, and show positive body language by facing the client and not hopping about on one foot ready to take off for an early lunch!

》 Get up and go!

Discuss with a colleague the effects of positive and negative body language when dealing with clients.

Attend to clients and enquiries (2)

Identifying the purpose of an enquiry

Not all visitors to the salon will be clients wanting to make an appointment. They may have come to make a delivery or to read the water meter. Whatever the nature of the enquiry, find out what the purpose is as soon as possible. If you are busy, acknowledge the person and indicate you will be with him or her shortly.

The enquiry could come from a telephone call. For example, it might be a technical rep who is new to the area needing directions to your salon. Locate a map of the local area showing where the salon is and keep it handy just in case you need to help someone find their way.

Should you need another member of staff to help you, inform the visitor you will not be long and seek further assistance promptly. An efficient, friendly manner will give a good first impression of how the salon deals with visitors by correctly identifying the purpose of the enquiry.

Confirming appointments

The salon's business is driven by those who operate the appointments system. Perhaps your salon has a manual system, where appointments are written in pencil in an appointments book, or there may be an electronic system (a computer). As soon as the client comes into the salon, ask how you can help and identify the client's appointment as efficiently as you can. Once you have confirmed their appointment, promptly inform the relevant member of staff. Suggest to your client, he or she might like to take a seat if they are early or if they have to wait for the stylist. This is also a good opportunity to practise your client-care policy by offering refreshments and magazines.

Some salons have a self-service touch-screen appointments system whereby clients can check themselves in on arrival. What advantages might a system like this have? Of course, there will be no crowding around the reception desk as clients who have booked appointments can use the screen and then make their own way to the waiting area where you can greet them personally and offer refreshments as usual. More and more businesses are realising the benefits of IT, and salons have reaped the rewards of using automated tills, appointment and stock systems for many years.

>> Get up and go!

Find out the costs of different treatments and services offered by your salon. Clients may ask you for this information when they make an appointment. Find out how long each treatment or service takes. What is your salon's procedure for making and recording appointments? Discuss your findings with your assessor.

? Memory jogger

Why is it important to make client appointments correctly?

The telephone is ringing and a client is also waiting at reception. In which order do you deal with the enquiries?

List four different enquiries a salon receptionist might deal with during a normal day.

A client would like an appointment with Sheila at 10.30 am but she is busy then. What could you do?

What items of stationery should be available at reception at all times?

Attend to clients and enquiries (3)

Recording messages

The importance of passing on messages to the right person at the right time often requires diplomacy and tact. You must be able to read the situation in the salon before rushing in to pass on a message. You will need to learn how and when to ask questions and to say things that suit the purpose of the call.

Below are some typical situations you may have to deal with.

- *The senior stylist is busy with a client. Her mum rings with an important message.* It is often best to check if the stylist is able to come to the telephone to take the call and, if not, write the message down.

- *A client has phoned to complain about a service she has received and has asked to speak to the manager.* In situations such as this, you will need to be calm, responsible and tactful. If the manager is not there or busy, tell the client the manager will call them back. Speak clearly to avoid any confusion and write down as much information as the client can give you, not forgetting their telephone number.

Show the client you have listened by recapping the information. This will also ensure you have all the correct information and there is no misunderstanding. Keep your tone of voice objective (i.e. don't take sides). Politely ask the client to hold, then take the message to a senior member of staff and await instructions.

When writing down a message, use your salon's message pad. Listen carefully to the caller before writing down the message. Always read it back to confirm accuracy. Take the message to the stylist or the person concerned and pass any reply back to the caller. Give all information clearly and accurately and make sure all confidential information is given only to authorised people.

Telephone Message

FOR: Ian
FROM: Mrs Price
TEL. NO.: 020 870181
TELEPHONED ✓   PLEASE RING ✓
CALLED TO SEE YOU ☐   WILL CALL AGAIN ☐
WANTS TO SEE YOU ☐   URGENT ☐
MESSAGE: Needs to speak to you asap – call on the above number up to 5.30pm
DATE: 29.09.09   TIME: 11.15am
RECEIVED BY: Robert

Use the salon's message pad to take down messages

» **Get up and go!**

What is your salon's policy for taking and recording messages? Discuss with a colleague what to do in each of the following situations:

- A client rings for a treatment list and tariff.
- The wholesaler rings to confirm the salon's order.
- A future bride is enquiring about the cost of three hair-up styles.

Confidential information

What is confidential information? In the salon, this will include:

- the contents of client records
- client and staff personal details such as name, address and telephone number
- financial matters relating to the business.

Sometimes personal conversations with colleagues may be confidential. Confidential information should only be given to authorised people.

The Data Protection Act (1998)

Under this act, you must not pass on any personal information to another person without the permission of the person involved. Your salon may obtain, hold and use personal data which is relevant for its own use. The consequences of dealing with confidential information inappropriately may lead to a disciplinary procedure. Take care only to use business information for the purposes of the business and keep the information within the walls of the salon.

» **Get up and go!**

Find out what your salon's procedures are for maintaining confidentiality. What might be the consequences if you break the salon's confidentiality policy?

Write down the differences between using an appointment book and a computer when making clients' appointments in relation to confidentiality.

? Memory jogger

A client is early for their appointment – what needs to be done?

A client is extremely annoyed because she has lost her earring at the salon. What can you do about it?

What is the main purpose of the Data Protection Act?

Why is it important to pass on messages at the time of receiving them?

Why is it important to have good communication between salon staff?

What type of answer can you expect from a closed question?

Help to make appointments for salon services (I)

People contact the salon in a variety of ways. It could be that clients telephone, visit the salon, a friend may make an appointment on their behalf, or they may send an email or text message to enquire about an appointment. You will need to know about the services the salon offers together with the products and available times you can offer an appointment.

Information such as each stylist's lunch hour, start and finish times, day off and late nights worked is all part of how your salon operates, and it will help you to know this when making appointments. Services such as cuts, blow-dries, sets, conditioning treatments and hair-up styles are non-chemical treatments. Colours, perms, relaxers, bleach, highlights and lowlights are chemical treatments. The salon will set aside a specific amount of time for each service. For example, it may take a few hours to complete a chemical service, while a cut or set may take less than an hour. You must make sure you leave enough time for each service to be finished professionally.

When making an appointment always make sure you deal with the request politely and promptly.

Page from an electronic appointments book

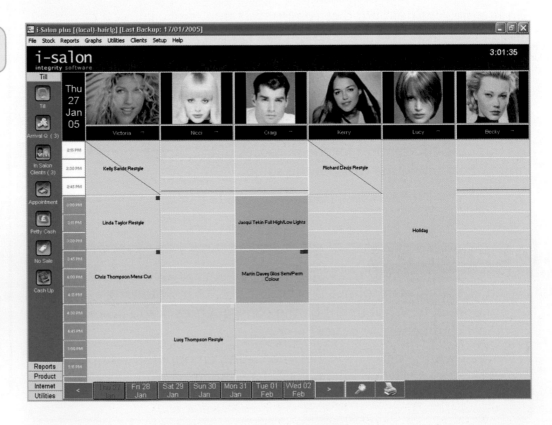

Identifying the client's requirements

Your client's request may take a few minutes to deal with and may cover a range of services offered by the salon. It's also possible the client may be making an appointment for several people and this will need your patience and knowledge of how the salon operates. Look at the appointment page and find out who is free and who will be able to offer each of the services requested. Ask for the client's name and the treatment they are interested in, enquire about the timeframe most suitable to your client and ask which member of staff they would like to carry out the treatment. Record their telephone number alongside their name in case there is a need to change the appointment. If you are not sure how to deal with a particular appointment request, then you should ask a senior member of staff for assistance.

Confirming appointment details

Your client's name, telephone number, service requested, date, time and member of staff booked for the service must always be discussed and confirmed with the client when he or she makes an appointment. Repeat the information for the appointment to the client and ask if it is acceptable. Always make sure the client is aware of the length of time anticipated for their particular treatment. If the client is in the salon, ask whether he or she would like an appointment card with the details written down.

On the appointment page or computer screen, make sure all of the information is recorded accurately, in the right place, at the right time and you have left the stylist sufficient time to complete the service. This means, for example, not booking a chemical treatment too late in the afternoon, as this would mean both stylist and junior stylist leaving the salon later than usual at the end of the day.

If using a manual appointment system, make sure your writing is neat and easy to read. Use a pencil to make appointments so that mistakes or cancellations can be easily changed. This helps to make good use of the available space on the page and keeps the information clear and easy to follow.

>> Get up and go!

With a colleague, practise making appointments for the following clients:

- Mrs McMillan would like a blow-dry. She has long hair.
- Mrs Gilchrist would like a perm and cut.
- Mr Griffen would like a dry cut.
- Miss Nicol would like highlights on medium-length hair.
- Mr Schneider would like a beard trim.

Help to make appointments for salon services (2)

Telephone appointments

Many appointments are made by telephone. When answering the phone, remember to smile – the client can hear the difference in your tone of voice! Listen carefully to what the client is saying and make each appointment as promptly as you can. Using the phone properly and efficiently is important to the smooth running of the salon business. It can be the first point of contact between you and the client.

On answering the phone, remember to tell the caller the name of the salon and who you are, for example 'Good morning, Head Start, Laura speaking. How can I help you?' As soon as the caller tells you his or her name, start to use it. It gives the call a personal touch and lets them know you have listened to basic information and as such, you have already begun to develop a professional relationship.

If you need to discuss appointment details with a colleague, it is a good idea not to leave the client holding on listening to salon background noise. Most phones have a mute button which will allow you to talk to your colleague without the caller hearing. Remember to press the mute button again when you return to speak to the client, otherwise he or she will not hear you! Repeat the information back to the client and check he or she is happy with the appointment time, date and stylist.

If you are making an appointment for a client who would like a permanent colour which touches the skin, you must remember to offer a skin test. Skin tests are recommended by the manufacturer and should be carried out 24–48 hours before the permanent colour application. Complete the appointment booking by saying something like, 'Thank you. We look forward to seeing you soon. Goodbye.'

This section is designed to further develop your skills and knowledge whilst working on reception. It will help familiarise you with how payments are handled. The most popular type of payment is cash, closely followed by credit or debit cards. Other types of payment include:

- cheques
- gift vouchers
- account.

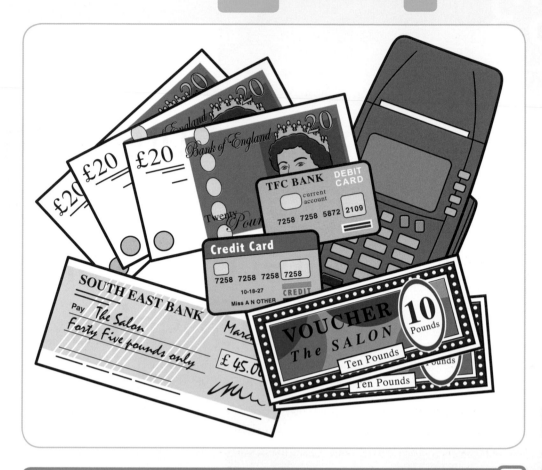

There are many different methods of payment

Get ahead

What do you need to be aware of when a client hands over money at reception? There are lots of forged notes and coins in circulation and you need to know how to deal with a situation where you think a client is trying to pay with forged money, should it arise. Talk to your assessor about the advantages and disadvantages of handling cash as opposed to credit and debit cards.

Draw up a simple SWOT chart and list the Strengths, Weaknesses, Opportunities and Threats of using cash and credit/debit cards. Compare these methods of payment with cheques, gift vouchers and payment by account.

Things for you to think about:

- Does your salon still accept cheques? Is a cheque guarantee card needed?
- Are credit/debit cards still valid? Check the expiry date.
- The cost to the salon of using credit/debit cards – banks charge businesses for this service.
- Are gift vouchers still valid? Always check the use-by date.
- Are accounts paid on time?

Memory jogger

List the information needed when making an appointment.

When the phone rings, how soon should you answer it?

When answering the phone, what should you say?

Give two reasons why appointments need to be made correctly.

What types of payment method does your salon accept?

UNIT G3

Contribute to the development of effective working relationships

Anne Veck, photographer: Clark Wiseman

A happy salon is a pleasant place to work and visit. Good working relationships with clients and colleagues are essential to the smooth running of the salon. A client's trust and goodwill must be earned. Showing you can do your job well will give clients confidence in your ability. If you upset a client or behave in an unprofessional way, the client may not come back to the salon. On the other hand, if the client is happy with your work, he or she is likely to return. You are very much a part of a team when you work in the salon.

This unit is about forming good relationships with clients in a way that promotes goodwill and trust, being able to work effectively when supporting your colleagues and using opportunities for learning within your job role.

In this unit you will learn how to:

- Develop effective working relationships with clients
- Develop effective working relationships with colleagues
- Develop yourself within the job role
- Understand employment policies and procedures.

This unit will also give you the chance to find out the best ways to develop your skills within your job role. You will then be ready to move on in your chosen career.

Here are some key

Communication – verbal and non-verbal ways in which to transfer information

Appeals procedure – a procedure you can follow should you have a grievance

Confidential – respect and privacy of an individual's information

Hospitality – offering refreshments, making the client comfortable

Courteous – polite and with good manners

Professional development – training activities to improve your skills/knowledge

Relevant person – responsible person

Technical activities – cutting, perming, colouring and straightening treatments

SWOT – Strengths, Weaknesses, Opportunities, Threats

TEAM – Together Everyone Achieves More

Goodwill – professional bond brought about by trust and respect

Trust – professional confidence

Develop effective working relationships with clients (I)

Clients are the most important part of your work. You will need to treat them with respect, which will help them to trust you and make them want to keep coming back. Welcome your client with a smile and by offering refreshments and magazines, making sure they are comfortable.

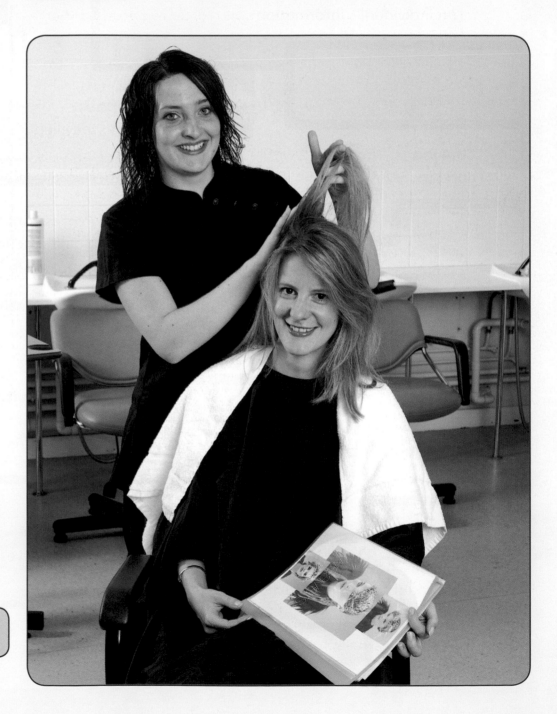

Listen carefully to what the client is saying

Communicating with clients

When communicating with your clients, try to remember the following.

- Use a friendly, calm, confident and polite manner.
- Try to attract and keep eye contact.
- Listen, and focus on what the client is saying.
- Use good questioning skills in order to find out information.
- Maintain client confidentiality by respecting them as people who trust you enough to carry out a professional treatment.
- Keep all you hear from your clients to yourself. Do not gossip, either about clients or to clients.
- Use positive body language. Stand up straight and use your eyes to express yourself when talking, remembering to smile. This will put the client at ease, especially if they are shy and timid.

Handling clients' personal items

Often clients will trust you to take care of their belongings while they visit the salon. Look in your reception area to see if there is a sign which makes it clear that the salon does not take responsibility for personal belongings, even if there is somewhere to hang coats and bags. Whatever your salon's policy for clients' belongings, it must be communicated clearly to them. Nevertheless, you should handle clients' belongings with reasonable care.

Dealing with client concerns

There are many mirrors in a salon and you will need to learn to use them for different purposes. Think about using the mirror to hold a conversation, or to look at the hairstyle as it is developing. You can also use the mirror to check for signs of unhappiness, or if the client is confused or angry. How would you recognise when a client is angry or confused?

To be an effective team member, you must make sure the client's comfort and needs are dealt with confidentially and professionally. It may be that the client's concern is within your job responsibilities, and you can deal with it in a professional way. Should you ever need to discuss a client's concern, you should know who to report the matter to. The salon manager is usually the person to report difficult situations to. Always work within your salon's client-care policy and deal with the concern promptly and efficiently. This will encourage the client's trust and goodwill.

Get up and go!

Clients who have cause to complain may do so quite loudly. This could lead to an embarrassing situation for all staff and clients in the salon. Remember to let the client know how their complaint is being dealt with and by whom. No one likes to be kept waiting, so deal with queries and concerns promptly. Does your salon have a complaints procedure? Is there a process to follow for client complaints? Research your salon for a policy on how to deal with a client complaint, finding out who deals with these issues. Consider how best to deal with a complaining client and make appropriate suggestions to your assessor.

Develop effective working relationships with clients (2)

Client comfort

Look after your clients. Offer them a drink and a magazine, and perhaps discuss other treatments or services the salon offers. Always offer them the same level of professionalism on each and every visit. Ask simple questions to make sure they are comfortable and to let them know you have thought about their comfort and care. Ask at regular intervals if they feel satisfied with the level of treatment they have received. You must strive to satisfy your client on every visit to ensure their return.

Your appearance and behaviour

Your standard of behaviour must be professional at all times. The way staff behave, either when dealing with clients or with each other, will be noticed by everyone in the salon. Remember, your behaviour contributes greatly to your professional image and this includes being punctual and having a good record of attendance.

The client's comfort is very important

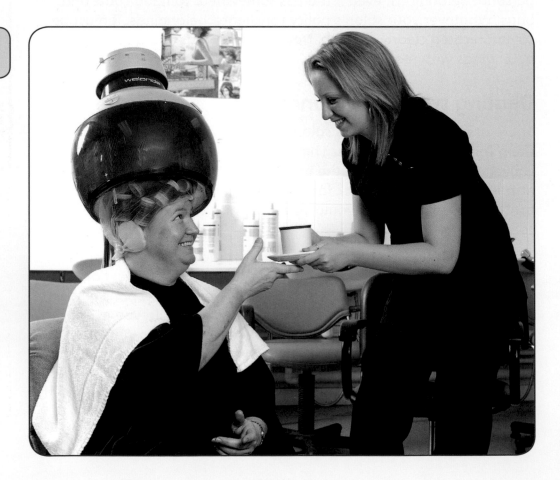

» Get up and go!

Manners cost nothing and yet they are one of the most important attibutes and will help you develop a good relationship with your clients and colleagues.

Try this: set yourself a target of giving and receiving at least ten 'thank yous' during your working day. Each time you do something for someone and they say thank you, jot it down and work towards your target of ten. How many times do you thank people? Now work towards your own target of giving ten.

This is a nice exercise and one which should be fun and easy to do. What's more, it should help you to realise how many times people recognise what you have done for them and, of course, remember that it is a two-way street.

Could you display this information discreetly on the salon wall, just to let people know you are developing your working relationships?

Know your salon's standards for appearance and meet them by wearing the appropriate uniform, make-up and jewellery. You will also need a suitable professional hairstyle. This must reflect your salon's standards and image, and will show clients you take pride in your own hair and appearance, helping you build a professional relationship with them.

Sharpen up!

Think about the different standards of dress within your salon and other places of work you have had contact with (e.g. shops, banks, other salons).

What did you think when you saw the staff? Were they suitably dressed? Did they look professional?

Consider these points and think about how your clients may view the staff who are attending to them, based on their appearance.

? Memory jogger

Who is responsible for your clients' belongings?

Think of three reasons why you should look after your client when they visit the salon.

How would you recognise that your client is angry or confused?

Why are attendance and punctuality important from a client perspective?

Develop effective working relationships with colleagues (I)

Teamwork is vital to the smooth running of the salon. You will need to be sure the people you work with are happy about how you are carrying out your job role. Unless you ask how well you are performing your role, possibly you will not find out until there is something to discuss, and then it may be from your line manager's point of view. Make general enquiries about how you are performing and whether you have done what has been asked of you on a regular basis.

You are an important member of staff who is central to the success of all treatments taking place within your salon. Your role is to help your team as much as you can, all day and every day. Your colleagues are relying on you to carry out your job in a professional way. Do not let them or your clients down by failing to turn up at work.

All staff need to be motivated and should aim to offer their clients a professional service. Good working relationships are important to the smooth running of the salon and all staff must be happy to take part in whatever job needs doing. Below is a simple acronym which will help you to remember what teamwork is all about:

Together
Everyone
Achieves
More

Being courteous

A happy salon environment makes a good impression on clients. Staff working well together – being friendly, helping each other and behaving like a team – will help to create a good atmosphere. As well as being friendly and respectful to clients, you must also be friendly and respectful to colleagues.

Asking for and giving help

When asking colleagues for help and information, you should be polite and courteous. Sometimes it is not what you ask for, but the way in which you ask for it that counts. If a colleague asks for your help, always give it willingly and with a smile.

Making efficient use of your time

Stylists and managers expect to receive a speedy and efficient service from their staff, which is you! You will need to manage your time well, which in turn will help the salon to run smoothly. In a salon, time is

---

» Get up and go!

Angela is a junior stylist at Richard's Salon. She finishes work at 6 pm. Below is a list of what Angela needs to do this evening by 11.30pm when she wants to go to bed. When you have read through the list, work out with a colleague how Angela can make the most effective use of her time by planning her evening. Don't forget to leave some time for a quick evening meal!

- Walk home – 10 minutes
- Read chapter of hairdressing book – 50 minutes
- Revise for a major exam – 40 minutes
- Work on project – 35 minutes
- Email boyfriend – 15 minutes
- Watch TV at 8.30 pm for 90 minutes
- Jog around park – 60 minutes

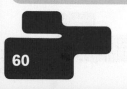

money so it is essential your time and your colleagues' time is used effectively. In practice, this means making sure everything is prepared ready for the stylist to move on to the next client.

Your line manager

There may be times when you need to speak to your line manager, either about work-related issues (e.g. treatments, procedures, policies) or other things, such as training, holiday or time off. Always treat a manager with the respect their position deserves. Managers have worked hard to achieve their job role and are in a good position to help you if you show them you are serious about your career. If you need time off, make sure you have a genuine reason and ask politely for their agreement, giving as much notice as possible.

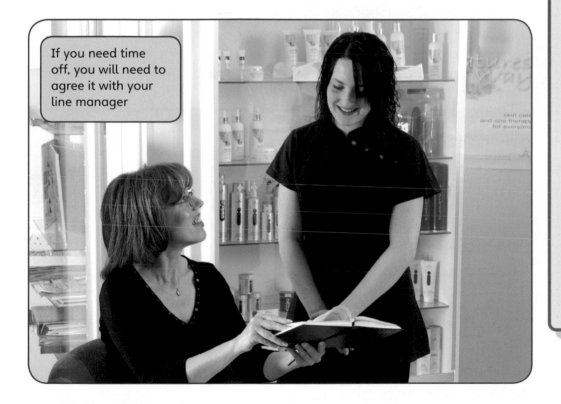

If you need time off, you will need to agree it with your line manager

>> **Get up and go!**

Look at the list of appointments below.

- Mrs Kraft – perm and set at 9.30 am
- Miss Wyatt – highlights and a cut at 10 am
- Mr Rossetti – beard trim at 11.30 am
- Miss Zhang – cut and blow-dry at 2.30 pm
- Mrs Morris – dry trim at 4 pm
- Mrs Cooper – hair up at 5 pm

Sue is a stylist who works from 9 am through to 6 pm. Create a stylist's column for Sue's day, blocking out the time needed to work on each client. For example, Sue will need 30 minutes to wind Mrs Kraft's perm, 15 minutes to set it and a further 15 minutes to dress out. Can Sue have lunch and, if so, when?

>> **Get up and go!**

With a colleague, take on the roles of line manager and salon junior and role play asking for an early lunch hour. The junior should use negative types of communication in the first instance and then try again using positive types of communication. How did the person playing the manager respond in both instances? Which approach do you think is best? Discuss the results of your scenario with your assessor.

Develop effective working relationships with colleagues (2)

Assisting colleagues

Your job includes passing tools and equipment such as rollers, pins, perm papers and perm rods to the stylist. You should pass these in such a way as to enable the stylist to progress more quickly with the treatment. This will help the stylist to make efficient use of their time.

Making drinks for clients, cleaning the backwash basins, sweeping the floor, maintaining record cards, carrying out skin tests, flushing the hot water through first thing in the morning, and replacing the barbicide are all part of your daily responsibilities. You can also assist colleagues by ensuring the reception area is clean and tidy and all retail shelves are neatly displayed and fully stocked. Keep the salon tidy by clearing away used towels, used cups and saucers, and tinting bowls, which will need to be rinsed out.

 Sharpen up!

Why not create a checklist to include your main tasks during the day? This checklist could include a column for tasks, a column for each hour of the day and a column for your initials. This way both you and your line manager will be able to keep an eye on when the tasks were last completed.

Some of the hands-on hair treatments you will be asked to do will include:

- shampooing
- colour removal
- neutralising
- conditioning treatments
- removing rollers and perm rods
- preparing clients' hair for further treatments, such as sectioning the hair so the stylist can apply colour.

Always give assistance to your colleagues which matches your job responsibilities.

» Get up and go!

Running out of products or other resources may seriously affect salon services. Always report any problems such as this to the relevant person. Who is this person in your salon?

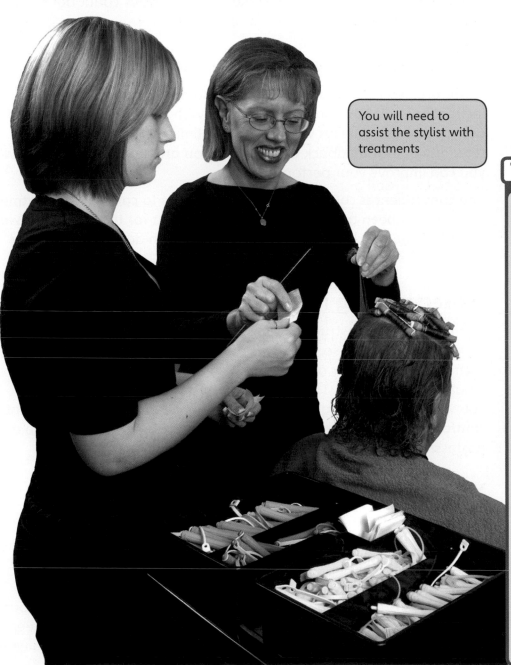

You will need to assist the stylist with treatments

? Memory jogger

How can you contribute to effective working relationships?

What teams are you part of? How do you feel when people do not play their part?

Discuss with a colleague how you would fit into an existing team.

How would you feel if you were trying to speak to someone and the person appeared bored or did not bother to look at you?

If you need time off, how do you ask your line manager's permission?

With a colleague, write a list of genuine reasons for taking time off from work.

Develop yourself within the job role (I)

Try to get into the habit of identifying your own strengths and areas for further improvement. On a regular basis you will have the opportunity to sit down with your line manager, or another person who is responsible for staff development, to agree an appropriate way forward for you to develop further in your job role. Use this opportunity positively, keep a record of what was discussed and consider any training you undertake as part of your continuous professional development.

Working within your responsibilities

If you are asked to do a task but are unsure how to do it or the instructions you have are unclear, check with your line manager about how to proceed. Always work within the limits of your job role and regularly ask for feedback on how well you are progressing and how you can improve your performance.

The consequences could be serious if you were to carry out a treatment you had not been trained to do. Use equipment for the purpose it was intended and check it is safe to use. If you are in doubt, ask a senior member of staff.

Understanding instructions

You may find the instructions you have been given to carry out a task are not clear. If so, discuss the appropriate course of action with a senior member of staff. This will ensure you know exactly what you have to do. The task can then be carried out correctly, you will avoid misusing a product or piece of equipment, and client comfort and satisfaction will be maintained, helping to promote a professional image.

Your professional development

How you develop in your job role is important to your own professional progression and to the success of the salon. By working with the person who is responsible for providing staff training in your salon, you will be able to develop your own personal training plan for success.

Using the existing framework of qualifications as a guide, make your plan. When you have developed your own professional record, keep it up to date. Many of your senior colleagues will be able to help with this as it is also part of their job to keep themselves up to date.

Discuss your personal training plan with your supervisor and plan how you are going to achieve areas for further development. Remember to include a review date when you can sit down together to review your progress.

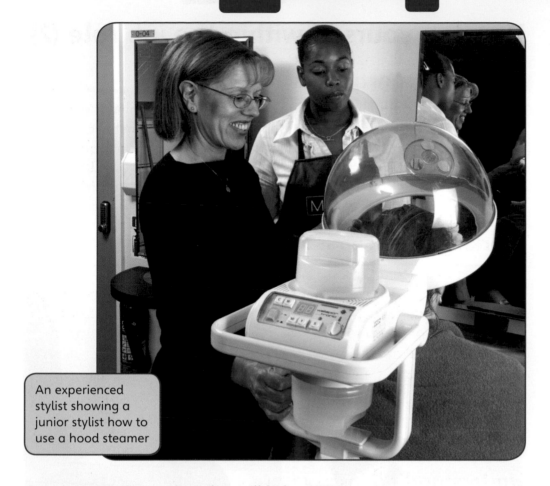

An experienced stylist showing a junior stylist how to use a hood steamer

Carrying out your action plan will help you to:

- develop your strengths
- focus on areas for further development
- promote good working relationships within the salon
- become more efficient at your job in the salon.

It is a good idea to keep a daily record of the type of work you do, so you and your manager can reflect on what you have been doing. It is best to have a weekly review so your memory is clear and a positive discussion can take place.

>> **Get up and go!**

Good staff are hard to find. What do you think are the qualities that make a good salon staff member? Make a list. Now list the types of things you want to improve, for example, your shampooing or communication skills. Think about the future. What do you want to achieve? Where do you want to be in five years' time? How are you going to get there? Discuss these questions with a colleague and develop a SWOT chart, listing your Strengths, Weaknesses, Opportunities and Threats.

Develop yourself within the job role (2)

Learning opportunities

Everyone learns differently. You may learn best by watching a stylist at work, or by listening to instructions either before or while you are doing a task. Take advantage of all the skills being demonstrated every day by senior staff. You can also learn when assisting stylists. Look at how they stand or hold their hands when carrying out a treatment. Look at the client's hair before, during and after the service so you can see how the style develops.

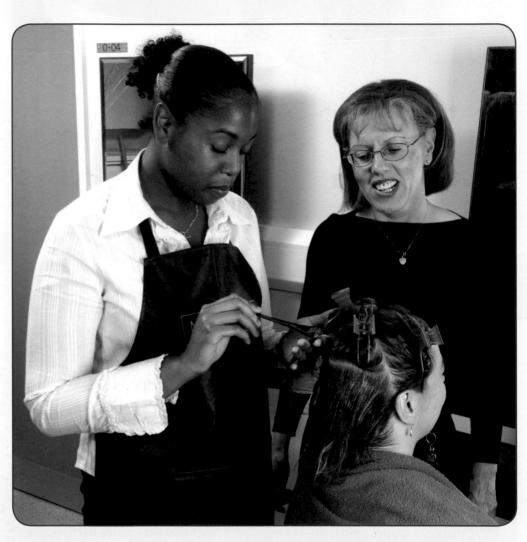

A junior stylist being trained to apply a conditioning treatment

There are many opportunities to learn and develop your professional skills. Try visiting some of the shows and exhibitions held every year to see top stylists demonstrate hair-up styles, cuts, colours and other new and exciting aspects of the hairdressing industry. Ask your colleagues to help you learn if you find tasks difficult and take advantage of opportunities to learn when they are available, e.g. late-night training sessions, guest stylists, trade reps, etc.

Watch some of the many TV channels showing hairdressing salons and the many and varied types of work they are involved in. Keep up to date with techniques and products by reading the weekly *Hairdressers Journal*. Look at pop stars, movie stars and so on to find out what the latest fashions and trends are. Hairdressing is all about fashion and you must be up to date. Attend each and every staff training session and take part in the salon's training and development plan. Watch technical services and ask questions about what you see and why it is happening.

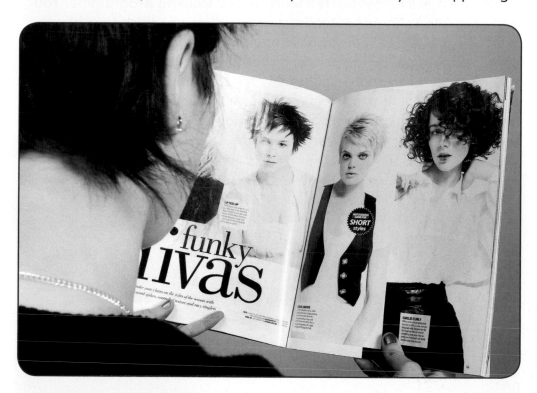

Magazines can help you keep up to date with trends and fashions in hairdressing

» Get up and go!

With a partner, role play an experienced stylist instructing a junior stylist on how to blow-dry using a handheld hairdryer. The junior can practise sectioning the hair and holding the hairdryer correctly. Think of the stages involved in training someone: planning, preparation, locating suitable resources, choosing an appropriate time to demonstrate, etc. Also consider the health and safety aspects.

Now write up an activity plan where the points mentioned above have been addressed. Enlist the help of a couple of colleagues and put your plan into action. Reflect on the practicalities of the before, during and after stages of the demonstration and write up your thoughts on improvements for a future training event. This exercise should help you develop an understanding of the amount of time, effort and work that goes into giving a demonstration. Did you use your people skills to best effect?

Develop yourself within the job role (3)

Setting self-development targets and reviewing progress

Many salons will expect you to achieve Level I within one year. It is possible to achieve this qualification within this time, which would then mean you could be considered for a Level 2 training programme. You and your salon should set realistic targets through which to achieve units of work. Agree realistic development targets for yourself with your line manager or the person responsible for staff development. You must take personal responsibility for your own targets and understand the importance of meeting them. The salon owner may be unhappy if you fail to do so! Your personal development plan must be used continuously for the rest of your life.

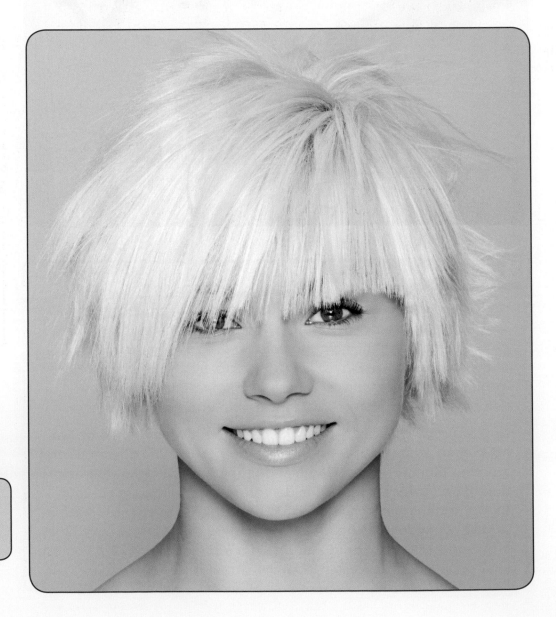

Professional development includes keeping up to date with the latest styles, techniques and products

A calendar showing progression and achievement would be a useful piece of evidence to develop. This should show clearly what you need to do and by what date. It could also set out the salon's commitment to you as a staff member in terms of training. Review your progress regularly with your manager and use this to develop any further action you may need in working towards your agreed targets.

Meeting your self-development targets should lead to increased job satisfaction, and the opportunity to progress to other areas within hairdressing and attract a higher financial reward.

>> **Get up and go!**

How can you identify your own strengths and areas for further development? Pair up with a colleague and jot down a few notes on how you are going to best identify these. How about a client questionnaire to provide you with feedback? Similarly, how about a simple feedback sheet to circulate amongst your colleagues at work? The questionnaire could be made anonymous so no-one feels uncomfortable about completing it. The findings from this exercise should be viewed positively, whatever they may be, and could form part of the review process.

? **Memory jogger**

How do you keep up to date with the latest styles, techniques and products?

How often does your salon hold team meetings to discuss general issues?

Why should you work positively within a team?

What might happen if you ignore manufacturers' or stylist's instructions?

Explain the benefits of continued professional development.

Why should you respond positively to reviews from staff?

Goldwell

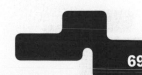

Employment policies and procedures

Procedures

Your job description and contract of employment

When you attend an interview, the job description (a list of the specific and general duties you will be expected to do) should be discussed. Once you start work at the salon, a copy of the job description will be placed in your records. Make sure you read it carefully and do what it says. You should be given a contract of employment within three months of starting your job.

Salon meetings

Most salons hold regular meetings and this is the time to discuss general issues which may concern you. Anything of a private nature must be kept confidential, such as staff details, client details, salon details and any disciplinary proceedings. Remember, if you breach the salon's policy for confidentiality, you could be disciplined.

The salon's appeals and grievance procedure

The salon will have copies of its appeals and grievance (complaints) procedure, which all members of staff should have access to. If you have a grievance, deal with the problem sensibly, calmly and professionally, and seek independent advice on how to deal with the situation. Find out who to report to when you have difficulties in working with a team member.

JOB DESCRIPTION – JUNIOR

Job title: Junior
Place of work: Styles 4 You, Paisley

Candidate specification
About the candidate
The candidate should:

- have good interpersonal skills and demonstrate a professional level of client care
- have the flexibility and willingness to work as a team member
- be able to work on Saturday and at least one late evening each week
- take responsibility for securing models for practise and assessment purposes
- update practical skills regularly at training sessions
- take an active interest in all aspects of work within the salon
- attend hairdressing seminars and professional courses in order to keep up to date with current and emerging techniques
- complete the appropriate hairdressing qualification within the specified time frame
- undertake other reasonable duties, from time to time, as required by senior staff.

Specific duties
Undertake day-to-day duties such as:

- shampoo and condition hair and scalp
- assist with perming, neutralising and colouring
- assist with salon reception duties
- sell retail products
- make refreshments
- reduce the risks to general health and safety
- sterilise equipment
- prepare hairdressing treatments and maintain the salon work areas (continuous)
- wash and dry towels and gowns
- check stock.

About the salon and our team
We are a friendly team who enjoy busy professional lives. We strive for perfection, sincerity and honesty in everything we do. Our skills are updated regularly by attending seminars and holding teach-in evenings. We look forward to working with you and wish you an enjoyable and rewarding time with us.

The successful candidate will enjoy: two weeks' paid holiday each year, the national minimum wage, a 37-hour working week, 9 am starts and one hour for lunch every day.

A job description for a salon junior

? Memory jogger

What may happen if you break rules of confidentiality?

Who would you report any problems in the salon to?

How can you identify your own strengths and areas for improvement?

Why should your salon have an appeals procedure?

UNIT GH3

Prepare for hair services and maintain work areas

Anne Veck, photographer: Clark Wiseman

When working in the salon, one of your main duties will be preparing clients for services and setting up products, tools and equipment for stylists. Regularly checking what services and treatments are booked, knowing what is needed for each of them and being able to tidy away and clean up properly afterwards are essential skills.

You will need to demonstrate that you can meet the standards for preparing and maintaining hairdressing work areas. Following certain health, safety and hygiene procedures will become a normal part of your day-to-day duties. Everything you have learned so far about health and safety and COSHH needs to be brought together in this unit. Go back to Unit G20 to remind yourself of the health and safety aspects of working in a salon. Your assessor will observe your performance, which must include preparation for different hairdressing treatments, such as ladies' or gents' hairdressing services.

In this unit you will learn how to:

- Prepare for hair services
- Maintain the work area for hair services.

Here are some key words you will meet in this unit:

Materials – resources you will need to carry out a client's treatment

Consultation – a meeting with a client to talk about and decide with them what they want from a treatment

Dispose – the correct removal of unwanted materials, products and other salon waste

Service – what you have given your client by way of your help, time and expertise, e.g. cut, blow dry, colour, perm, etc.

Stock – products, materials and resources needed for clients' treatments

Records – client details held either manually (on paper) or electronically (on computer)

Prepare for hair services (1)

Start as you mean to go on

Preparing for hair services isn't just about getting tools and equipment ready. Think about the type of people who may come through your salon door. Are they busy working people with little time on their hands? Are they parents with young children? Are they able-bodied or disabled? Notice your clients' body language as they enter the salon. Do they look rushed, frustrated, or perhaps calm?

You can begin to prepare for a client's hair service as soon as they enter the salon. If you notice a client has difficulty walking or moving around, or has a pushchair or shopping bags, find out if they need help coming into the salon. You may be able to hold the door for them, move things out of their way, or help them to a chair. Try to remember what help your client needed so you can be ready to offer it again next time they visit. Demonstrate a patient, positive attitude and make sure your body language is always professional.

» Get up and go!

Here are a few different services and treatments your salon may have booked on a regular basis:

Service/treatment	Products, tools and equipment needed
Setting	
Blow-drying	
Perming	
Colouring	
Cutting	
Straightening	
Hair-up	
Plaiting	
Hair extensions	
Shaving	
Beard trimming	

Copy out the table and for each service list in the right-hand column the products, tools and equipment that will be required. Don't forget things like cotton wool, disposable gloves and barrier cream, and whether or not you will need to set up a trolley.

Now practise setting up trays with a colleague. Check each other's trays and find out if you have both included everything you need.

Setting up materials, tools and equipment

Think about the most sensible way in which to set up materials, tools and equipment for the hair services offered by your salon. What clients do you have booked in today? You will need to check the appointment book, see what stock is required for each service and check you have the necessary items in the stock room. Discuss each client's requirements with your stylist.

Gowns and towels, and tools and equipment required for popular hairdressing treatments, must always be readily available. This will present a professional image and help save time for you and the stylist. The client will also be able to have their treatment completed in good time, making the visit a cost-effective one for the salon and an enjoyable one for the client.

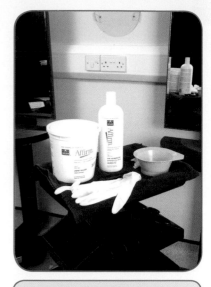

Preparing products and equipment for stylists is one of your most important responsibilities

As each of the services your salon offers has its own particular requirements in terms of resources, you need to be thorough in your preparation. It is particularly important to check all electrical equipment is in good working order, clean and fit for its purpose. Similarly, are products good to use? Check for any punctures or leaks in tubes and containers, and whether lids have been replaced properly. For example, the stylist will need the following if a perm is booked:

- disposable gloves
- plastic apron
- combs
- section clips
- different sized rods
- end papers
- cotton wool
- tension strips
- plastic cap
- barrier cream
- the appropriate perming lotion and neutraliser
- manufacturer's instructions.

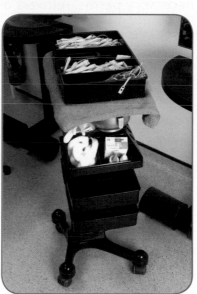

Perming trolley set up ready for stylist

[?] Memory jogger

What types of people may come through your salon door?

How do you know what to set up for each treatment your salon offers?

Prepare for hair services (2)

Preparing in good time

The tools, equipment and work area that stylists use need to be ready in time for the required treatment. Constantly think ahead and prepare the area as necessary for your stylist and, ultimately, your client. Be alert for signs that your team may need something, such as a comb or pair of clippers. Watch what each staff member uses – he or she may have a favourite comb or brush. Does this need to be sterilised before the next client?

Look at the appointment book on a regular basis so that you know what work is planned for the day. Bear in mind appointments might change during the day and you need to know the status of the appointment book at any one time. This means you need to liaise constantly with the receptionist to make sure changes are being passed on to you.

Now think about the type of work that has been booked in for the day. There may be several perms, some colours, a relaxer and a conditioning treatment. You will need to prepare for each treatment separately. Sometimes it is a good idea to check the appointments the day before, especially with chemical treatments. Check you have the necessary perms, relaxers and colours required for each of the clients.

Observe and anticipate

As you become more knowledgeable about hairdressing skills and get to know your colleagues, you will be able to observe what is happening in the salon and anticipate when your help is needed. Observation plays a major part in many hairdressing salons. Staff can 'speak' to each other using eye contact rather than words. Be alert to the signs that you may be needed and learn to identify your team's body language. This will help you anticipate the needs of other people, which in turn will benefit both clients and colleagues. Remember though to observe, not stare! Make sure that when you watch someone it is for a professional purpose.

At the end of a treatment

Timing in the salon is everything – sometimes things can happen too soon or not soon enough. Think about the products that may be needed at the end of a treatment. It could be serum, hairspray, wax, or a mixture of different products. Be on the look out for opportunities to assist your team as they are finishing off their clients.

Client records

Record cards are a professional record of what has been applied to your clients' hair. They are also a useful tool for recording positive comments and suggestions for any future treatment the client may request. The personal and professional information held on the record

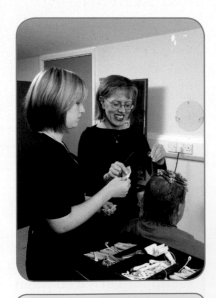

Be ready to hand tools, equipment or materials to the stylist when they need them

card is protected by the Data Protection Act. It is very important for record cards to be stored correctly in a lockable cabinet.

When obtaining records for your stylist's client, always remember to check the name, address and telephone number. Clients may share the same surname and even the same first name, and you don't want to give the stylist the wrong information.

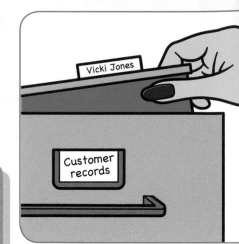

Clients' record cards must be stored properly in a locked cabinet

Sharpen up!

Client record cards hold detailed information from past treatments. This information is crucial to the success of any hairdressing treatment. Imagine a situation where a stylist is off sick. Would another stylist know what was previously used on the client? Do you remember all of the products, mixes, timings and results from past clients?

Records are important, to both your salon and your clients. They inform you of the products used previously, the timing and what the client's thoughts were regarding the result. Always have the client's record card ready in time for the consultation by the stylist. Clear away and file record cards as soon as they have been finished with. Your next client does not want the previous client's colour applied to his or her hair.

⟫ Get up and go!

Think of a retail incentive scheme where all staff are encouraged to sell retail products and more chemical and non-chemical treatments. This could lead to greater income for the salon and perhaps a higher return for all staff in terms of an increased salary.

Look at the retail chart below and think of a way in which all staff could benefit, from the junior to the senior manager.

Staff name	Week 1	Week 2	Week 3	Week 4
Sylvia				Straighteners
Sue	Conditioning mousse	Moisturising shampoo	Scrunchie	
Jane		Brush	Serum	
Charmaine	Hair shine		Chemical treatment	

At the end of week 4, the salon could simply total the cost of sales and reward the member of staff who sold the most. Some hairdressing companies donate gifts as retail incentives. Discuss this system with a senior member of staff at your next staff meeting.

? Memory jogger

Why is timing important when setting out materials and products for your stylist?

What could you check against to find out what stock is needed for the day ahead?

Where should record cards be kept?

What does 'confidential' mean?

For whose benefit are record cards kept?

Prepare for hair services (3)

Cleaning the work area and sterilising tools and equipment

Remember to clear away all materials, tools and equipment when the stylist has finished with them. Wipe down the styling area with a suitable cleansing liquid at the most appropriate time and make sure the area is hair-free. Think about how you would feel if a stylist used a comb on your hair that had been used on clients all day without being cleaned and sterilised.

Salons are breeding grounds for bacteria. Make sure all equipment is clean for every client. Combs, brushes and all tools and equipment that have come into contact with the client's hair and scalp must be cleaned and sterilised ready for the next client. Sterilising destroys all living organisms. You may also use disinfectants in the salon to clean work areas. Disinfecting slows down the growth of bacteria.

Methods of sterilisation

Different tools and equipment need to be sterilised using different methods. For example, soft plastics cannot withstand the heat of an autoclave (which reaches 125°C) and will change shape or simply melt – a plastic roller will come out looking like a chewed piece of gum! Be careful to choose the right method for each piece of equipment. Take advice and guidance from the stylist or senior manager on how to sterilise correctly.

The three most commonly used methods of sterilising salon tools and equipment are:

- barbicide
- ultraviolet cabinet
- autoclave.

Barbicide is often used for sterilising combs and scissors and should be changed daily. An ultraviolet cabinet can sterilise small pieces of equipment made of plastic, such as brushes, combs and section clips. Autoclaves will sterilise objects made of rubber and metals, such as good quality combs and scissors.

Get up and go!

Make a list of the different types of sterilisation methods available in your salon.

Find out how each one works and what tools they are used to sterilise.

Sharpen up!

What happens during a day in the life of a hairdresser? Think about your working day from start to finish and all the things you do. Many of them you probably do automatically and don't even think about. Maybe some of your colleagues aren't aware of all the things you do and how varied they are.

Make a list of all the tasks you do on an average day. Look at the list and think about how important each task is to the smooth running of the salon. Some of the things you do may be mundane, but if you didn't do them, life in the salon for your colleagues would soon become difficult.

Why not discuss your list at your next review or staff meeting? You may enlighten some people about what you do and ultimately surprise them!

? Memory jogger

What is the difference between disinfecting and sterilising?

Name three methods of sterilisation used in a salon.

What temperature does an autoclave reach?

Maintain the work area for hair services (I)

Disposing of hair and waste materials safely

The correct disposal of hair and waste materials is vital to the success of your salon. This isn't just to keep the salon looking clean and tidy – an Environmental Health Officer can, and often does, close down salons where staff have failed to deal with salon waste correctly.

Removing hair and waste from the salon means following health and safety procedures and using controlled and environmentally friendly methods. Here are some aspects of waste management you should be aware of.

- Loose hair should be cleared from basins to prevent blockages.

- Empty conditioner or shampoo bottles should be put in a plastics bin.

- Any left-over tint, bleach or perm lotion should be poured down the basin.

- Cut hair from the salon floor should be incinerated (burned) and disposed of by the local authority.

- Sharp items such as razor blades should be stored in a sharps box, which is then disposed of by a specialist company.

- Hairspray and mousse containers must be disposed of by a recognised company.

Removing waste quickly and correctly will give clients a professional image of the salon. It also reduces the risk of injury and cross-infection by keeping your work area clean and tidy during the service.

The Control of Substances Hazardous to Health (COSHH) Regulations (2002)

The COSHH Regulations greatly affect the way in which salons dispose of their waste by setting out basic measures employers and employees must take. In addition, each local authority has its own policy on how to deal with salon waste and this may mean that some salons have different procedures to others. However, in general, hair should be incinerated, aerosols should be disposed of separately from the general salon waste and sharps should be collected by a specialist refuse company.

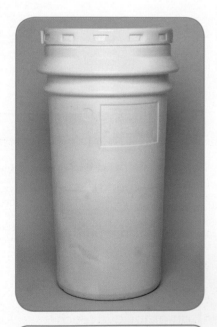

A sharps bin is the only way to dispose of items like razor blades

» Get up and go!

Look at the methods of waste disposal your salon adopts. How do they dispose of hair, plastics, aerosols, chemical products and sharps? Contact your Environmental Health Services department via your local authority to find out how to dispose of salon waste in the correct way. You can also ask your assessor about the different strategies in place that aim to minimise the effects on the environment of salon waste disposal. Have there been any changes or updates to best practice? Present your findings to your assessor.

Checking and cleaning equipment

All salon equipment must be checked visually before each use and cleaned after each use in readiness for the next client. Make sure equipment is cleaned thoroughly following the manufacturer's instructions. Remember to wear suitable personal protective equipment (PPE) if using chemicals or cleaning fluid. Electrical equipment should be checked by a qualified electrician and PAT (Portable Appliance Test) tested each year. This will satisfy any health and safety checks your salon has.

Floors, seating, working surfaces, mirrors and basins must also be cleaned on a daily basis using appropriate cleaning equipment. Depending on how big your salon is, you may have independent cleaners who clean on a regular basis.

Towels and gowns

To avoid cross-infection, it is very important that clean towels and gowns are used for each client. Cross-infection is when an infection (such as a cold) or an infestation (such as head lice) is passed from one person to another. Make sure you have clean gowns and towels for every treatment.

As mentioned earlier in the unit, regular checking of the day's appointments will help you plan ahead. You will need to find out how many chemical and non-chemical treatments are booked in for the day so you can ensure you have the appropriate number and colour of clean towels for each client. At the start of each day, make sure there are enough clean towels and gowns to last. This part of your work is very important – if there are not enough clean towels and gowns, your salon cannot carry out services and treatments!

? Memory jogger

Why is it important to dispose of salon waste safely and correctly?

What are your salon's waste management procedures?

What are sharps?

What does PAT stand for?

What needs to be cleaned in the salon every day?

Maintain the work area for hair services (2)

Stock

Stock is all the products, such as shampoo, conditioner, hairspray, colour, perm lotion, etc., and consumable equipment, such as hair grips, end papers, etc., that your salon needs to run smoothly. Stock-taking systems vary from salon to salon. It is your responsibility to make sure that no product falls below the minimum stock level and these levels will need to be monitored on a regular basis. The stylist or senior manager will advise you on how much stock needs to be kept for each item.

> **>> Get up and go!**
>
> Think about how it might be possible to improve the stock system at your salon. You could suggest a computerised system if the salon currently uses a manual one. If this isn't possible, why not come up with some improvements for the current system, such as using differently coloured pieces of paper to indicate how urgently ordering is needed or to list items that need ordering from different suppliers? Is this something you could discuss at one of your staff meetings?

Computerised stock systems

Your salon might have a computer system which updates stock levels as you enter sales. The system may also contain other information about the salon such as clients' records and details of each stylist's income and retail sales.

Storing stock

Make sure you know how and where to store materials, tools and equipment within your salon. Your responsibilities under the current COSHH Regulations are important when handling hair products and cleaning and disinfecting/sterilising chemicals. Some items of stock will need to be stored in a locked cabinet at ground level because of the chemicals they contain, including hydrogen peroxide, straightening products, bleaching, perming and neutralising products, and certain cleaning and disinfecting materials.

Consider your salon stock room and how the stock is stored. Ideally, nothing should be stored above head height, and all heavy items, such as large containers of shampoo and conditioner, should always be stored on the floor. Everything should be tidy and easy to find. Stock rotation should be practised so that older items are used before new ones.

Be knowledgeable about the stock your salon uses. Know what each product and item is for and how it should be used properly. Use personal protective equipment as appropriate when handling, storing or disposing of certain items.

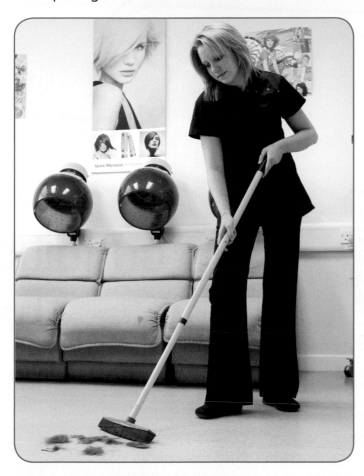

Floors will need to be swept throughout the day

Cleaning work surfaces

Cleaning work surfaces effectively and leaving them ready for further treatments should include not just the parts of the salon used by clients, but the areas where you mix and prepare chemicals and make drinks. The floor, reception seating area, all working surfaces and mirrors must be kept hygienically clean. Any spillages on the floor must be cleared away immediately. Remember to wear personal protective equipment if necessary.

Floors will need to be swept throughout the day and mopped at the end of each day with a suitable disinfectant. Mirrors should be wiped with a suitable glass cleaner to avoid smearing and all working surfaces must be cleaned with a bactericide. To minimise cross-infection, it is essential to follow good housekeeping practices at all times.

Health and safety laws require salons to keep their refreshments area separate from areas where chemicals are mixed or disposed of. This is essential to good hygiene and a professional standard of working.

? Memory jogger

What types of item need to be stored in a locked cabinet?

Why is it important to regularly check stock levels?

Why should you not make a client's drink in the same area you use for mixing hair products?

UNIT GH1

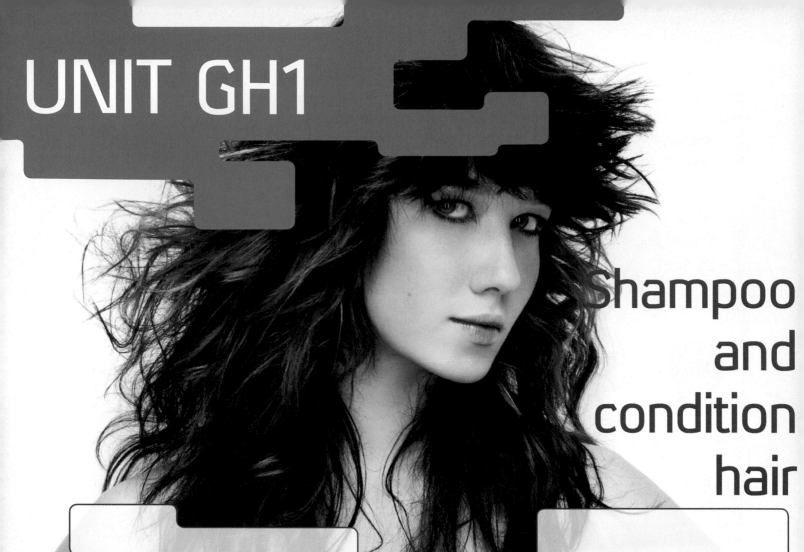

Shampoo and condition hair

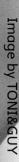

The word 'shampoo' is a Hindustani word meaning 'to press or rub'. Shampooing and conditioning hair is one of the most important treatments in hairdressing. It prepares the hair for any treatments or services and can be the start of a pleasurable hairdressing experience for the client – or a complete disaster if carried out incorrectly!

This unit is about the skill of shampooing and conditioning the hair and scalp. You will learn about different massage techniques and some of the products available for different hair types. This unit applies to both ladies' and gents' hairdressing salons.

In this unit you will learn how to:

- Maintain effective and safe methods of working when shampooing and conditioning hair
- Shampoo hair
- Apply and remove conditioners.

Here are some key words you will meet in this unit:

Minimise – reduce the effect of something

Friction – fast rubbing technique with a light plucking action

Products – shampoos, conditioners, styling sprays, creams and gels, etc.

Massage – manipulating the skin either manually or mechanically

Temperature – how hot or cold something is

Relevant person – assessor, stylist or line manager

Effleurage – slow, stroking, superficial movement, using the length of the hand

Rotary – penetrating, circular movement using the fingertips

Petrissage – slow, deep, penetrating circular movement using the fingertips

Surface – conditioner which lies on the outer layer of the hair shaft

Penetrating conditioner – conditioner which penetrates into the cortex layer of the hair shaft

Steamer – equipment providing moist heat, used during conditioning

Dermatitis – inflammation of the skin caused by an irritant

Maintain effective and safe methods of working when shampooing and conditioning hair (I)

Most people can shampoo their own hair at home and are likely to have done so many times. As a practising hairdresser, you will need to make sure your shampooing technique is of a high professional standard, and this will probably be a little different from how most people shampoo their own hair at home. The physical action of massaging a person's head can be invigorating, stimulating and relaxing. Be conscious of the person at your fingertips. Ask them how they like their hair and scalp to be shampooed.

Why shampoo hair?

We shampoo hair for three reasons.

- To remove excess natural oil, skin cells, dust and dirt.
- To remove the build-up of hair-care products.
- To prepare the hair for further treatments.

The success of the shampoo is important to the success of the following treatment, for example, the client's cut, perm or colour.

›› Get up and go!

Look at the various shampoos and conditioners in your salon. Now complete the table below matching the products in your salon with the hair types. This information will be useful when offering clients professional advice about their hair and scalp condition.

Hair/scalp type	Shampoo	Conditioner
Coloured	Colour preserver	Colour preserver
Fine		
Permed		
Normal		
Dry/damaged		
Dandruff-affected		
Oily		

Preparation

Your salon's requirements for client preparation should include a thorough hair and scalp analysis by an experienced stylist who will confirm whether it is safe for you to carry out the treatment.

Protecting the client

The client's clothing must be protected at all times. Always use a clean gown and towel. If the client is not gowned properly, their clothing may get wet, or even damaged if they are having a chemical treatment.

Positioning the client and checking your posture

Position the client correctly at either the backwash or front-wash basin and check your client is comfortable. The client's position will affect how you stand at the basin and how tired you will feel at the end of the shampoo. Poor posture may have a long-term effect on your wellbeing, so make sure your position and posture during the shampoo minimises the risk of tiredness and injury to yourself.

>> **Get up and go!**

Practise preparing a colleague for a shampoo with a gown, towel and a waterproof cape. Consider how claustrophobic it may make you feel if everything is too tight. Remember to allow some room for your client to breathe – it can get warm under those protective layers. Always ask the client if they are comfortable.

Now find out how to prepare a client for the following services and practise on your colleague: perming; relaxing; colouring; cutting; setting.

? Memory jogger

Why do we shampoo hair?

What are the effects of having poor posture whilst shampooing your clients?

What products would you recommend for a client who has oily hair?

Why should you always gown a client correctly before carrying out any treatment?

What should be carried out before any hairdressing treatment begins?

What products would you recommend for a client with dry hair?

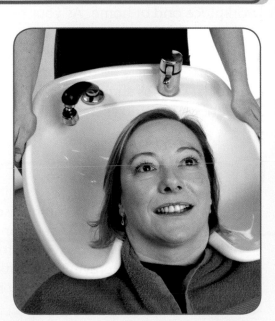

Position the client comfortably at a backwash basin

Maintain effective and safe methods of working when shampooing and conditioning hair (2)

Working methods

Using resources efficiently

Resources such as hairdressing products are expensive and it is important to use them cost effectively. Some shampoos have pump dispensers and these may help to reduce unnecessary waste by dispensing just the right amount of product. By minimising waste you save money, therefore making the salon a more profitable business.

Reducing the risk of cross-infection

Any tools or equipment that come into contact with clients' hair and skin must be completely clean. This will help to maintain a safe and hygienic working environment. As well as keeping the salon clean, you must always remember your personal cleanliness. Make sure your own standards of health and hygiene help to reduce the risk of cross-infection. For example, do not come into the salon if you have a cold or contagious disease, or an infestation such as head lice. Stay at home and minimise the risk of cross-infection; when the condition has cleared, it is then safe to return to work. By ensuring your personal standards of health and hygiene you minimise the risk of cross-infection, infestation and offence to your clients and colleagues.

Reducing the risk of injury

Your hands are essential to carrying out everyday tasks both in the workplace and at home. As your hands will often be in water, always dry them thoroughly and use a barrier cream and protective gloves. This will help to reduce the risk of contact dermatitis, a skin condition which often affects hairdressers. It is caused by constant contact with products, such as shampoos and chemicals. Should the condition worsen, you should seek medical advice.

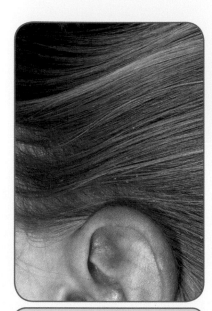

Head lice hatch from eggs called nits. They can be found on the hair shaft close to the scalp

>> Get up and go!

Next time you are in the salon, discreetly observe how many staff are wearing jewellery on their hands. It is best to leave your rings at home. This will make it easier for you to clean your hands properly and help prevent dermatitis. Ask your colleagues if they have ever suffered from dry, itchy hands or dermatitis.

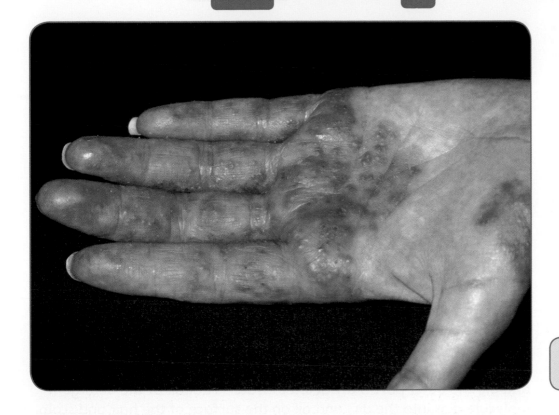

Protect your hands against dermatitis

It is essential to store, use, handle and dispose of products in accordance with manufacturers' instructions, salon policy and local bylaws. When dealing with resources in the salon, you will be expected to have a good working knowledge of the Control of Substances Hazardous to Health (COSHH) Regulations, therefore minimising the risk of harm or injury to yourself and others.

Re-filling and re-ordering products

Shampoos, conditioners and chemical products are in constant use in the salon.

Keep a look out for opportunities to replenish low levels of resources, when required, to minimise disruption to your own work and to clients. Should you notice that the stock level of any product is running low and needs re-ordering, report it to the relevant person.

» Get up and go!

With a colleague, think of reasons why shampoo and conditioner dispensers need to be regularly filled up and why stock levels of products need to be checked regularly. What might the effects be if the salon runs out of something? Who should stock shortages be reported to in your salon?

? Memory jogger

What are the appropriate measures for disposing of chemicals in the salon?

Why should you re-fill products on a regular basis?

What does COSHH stand for?

Describe how dermatitis can be prevented.

How can you use resources cost-effectively?

Shampooing hair (I)

How long should a shampooing and conditioning treatment take?

Depending on the length and thickness of the client's hair, a basic shampoo and surface condition should take 3–5 minutes. You might find it helpful to watch your colleagues and time them, making sure they make effective use of their working time. You must practise with:

- above shoulder-length hair
- below shoulder-length hair.

How shampoo works

Shampoo comes in many types, consistencies, colours and aromas. It mixes easily with water allowing grease, dirt and oil to be rinsed out of the hair. It works because it contains detergent molecules. Each detergent molecule consists of two parts – one part is attracted to dirt and oil, the other part is attracted to water. The tail of the detergent molecule digs into the dirt and oil on the surface of the hair and scalp. The head of the detergent molecule has a negative electric charge. As a result of massage movements, dirt and oil is repelled from the hair and rinsed away in the water.

How detergent molecules in shampoo cleanse the hair

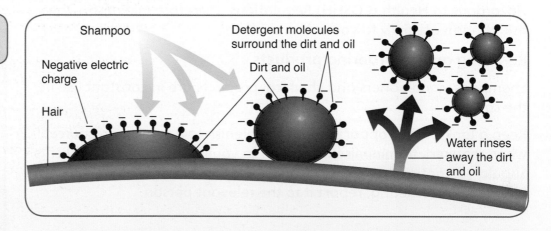

Shampoo flattens the surface tension of the water

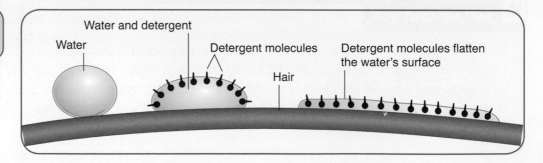

Water also has a high surface tension, which has the effect of producing a 'skin' on the surface of the water. Shampoos flatten the surface tension of water making it easier to shampoo the client's hair.

How conditioner works

Hair is made of a protein called keratin. The same protein is found in skin and nails.

Hair in poor condition may have been damaged by overuse of heated styling equipment, incorrect brushing or too many chemical treatments. Conditioners strengthen and moisturise the hair.

There are many types of conditioner. They include the following:

- Surface conditioner coats the hair shaft and smoothes down the cuticle scales leaving the hair tangle-free.

- Anti-oxidant conditioner prevents any further oxidation to the hair shaft after chemical treatments.

- Specialist treatment conditioners strengthen the hair shaft internally by filling the air spaces caused by damage with liquid protein. This gives the hair added elasticity, sheen and manageability.

- Almond or olive oils are used mainly for dry scalps.

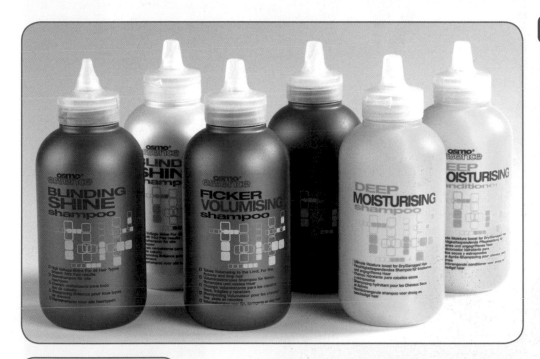

A range of conditioning shampoos

? Memory jogger

How long should a shampoo and conditioning treatment take to complete?

Briefly explain how shampoo works.

What protein is hair made from?

What might cause hair to become damaged?

Why might you use an almond or olive oil to treat hair?

Shampooing hair (2)

Working with the stylist

There are many different levels of staff within a salon, including:

- staff who shampoo and carry out basic skills
- staff who practise technical skills like perming, relaxing, cutting and colouring
- senior staff who may manage the salon.

An experienced stylist instructs a junior member of staff

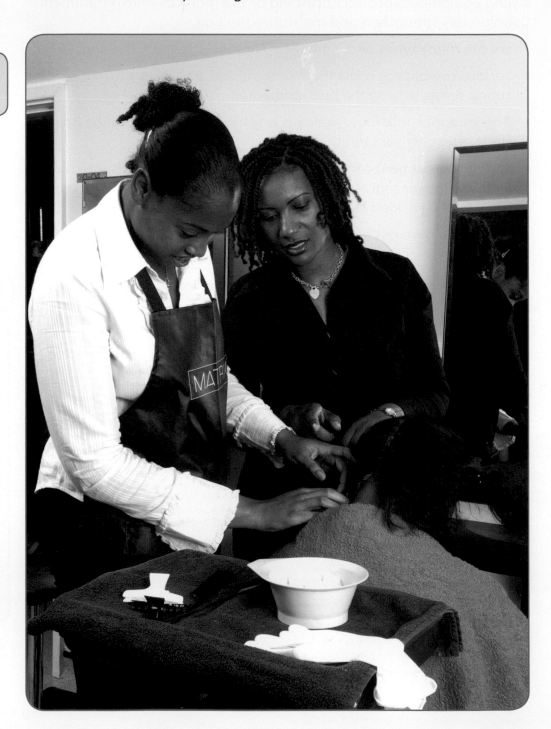

Part of your job role will involve learning to work with people and take instructions from senior colleagues. They may ask you to use a product in a particular way, or to change your massage movements to suit a different hair type and length. Following their advice and listening to the information they give will help you develop within your job role.

Using products and tools

Acid and alkali products

Acid and alkali products are regularly used in the salon. Acid products include perms, colours, shampoos, conditioners, bleach and peroxide. Acid-based conditioners are considered to be kinder to the hair because they close down the cuticle scales and return the pH of hair to pH 4.5–5.5. They also help maintain moisture within the hair shaft and give a smooth, shiny, tangle-free finish to the hair.

Alkali products include bleach, colours, perms, relaxers and some shampoos. These products lift the cuticle scales and give a roughened feel and appearance to the outer layer of the hair shaft. The pH of most hair when chemically treated is often more than pH 7, which is why the hair must be returned to its natural acid state of pH 4.5–5.5.

Steamers

A steamer produces a constant amount of steam contained within a hood. The hood is similar to that of a hood hairdryer. It works rather like a kettle. You will use a steamer to help:

- the penetration of conditioner
- replace lost moisture
- strengthen the internal and external layer of the hair shaft.

You should only use a steamer if you have been trained in how to do so and, as with all salon products, you should always follow the stylist's instructions in accordance with the manufacturer's instructions. The Electricity at Work Regulations cover the safe use of electrical equipment in the salon, including steamers (see Unit G20 for more information on these regulations).

First, fill the reservoir with distilled (not tap) water. This is to make sure no impurities coat the element and block the tiny water valves. With dry hands, plug in and switch on the steamer. While you massage the client's hair and scalp, the water will heat up and release steam into the hood. Place the client under the hood for 5–10 minutes. Remember to offer the client a drink or a magazine to read. When the time is up, take the client out from under the steamer. Switch off and unplug the steamer. Clean the steamer as soon as you have finished with it, leaving it ready for the next client.

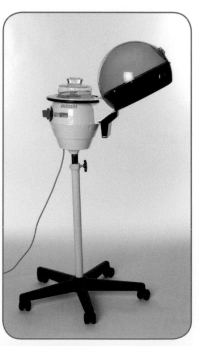

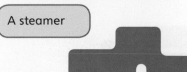
A steamer

Shampooing hair (3)

Water temperature and flow

The temperature of the water plays an important part in cleansing the hair and scalp. The flow of water is important too. Both the temperature and flow you use will depend on the amount of hair the client has and the sensitivity of their scalp. Very hot water will burn the client's scalp, but if the water is not hot enough, the hair will not be fully cleansed. There are times when you may need to use tepid (warm) water. For example, if the client's hair and scalp are oily, tepid water will help the sebaceous glands to produce less sebum (oil) when carrying out a light massage during the shampoo.

Test the temperature and flow of the water before you apply it to your client

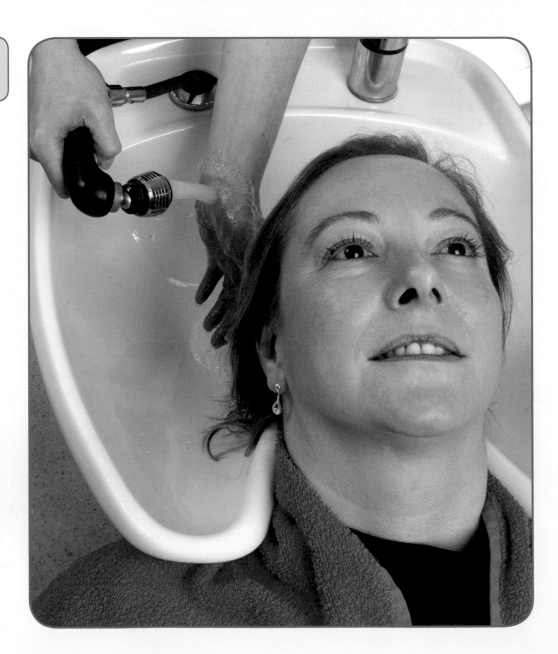

Before and during each shampoo, it is essential to test the temperature of the water, either on the back of your hand or on the inside of your wrist. Remember to check the temperature of the water is comfortable for your client regularly. Adapt the water temperature, flow and direction to suit the needs of your client's hair and the next part of the service. Always turn the tap off between shampoos. Hot water is too expensive to simply let run down the plughole!

Choosing shampoo

You will need to choose the most appropriate shampoo for the client's hair and scalp condition. Some treatments that follow a shampoo may not need a conditioner. For example, when perming a client's hair, conditioner will coat the cuticle and act as a barrier, giving an unsatisfactory result. Make sure you know which shampoo to use (go back to the table you completed on page 86 to remind yourself).

Be careful not to spill shampoo, but if you do, you will need to clear up any spillages straight away for the safety of your client, colleagues and yourself.

Get up and go!

Take a look at the different hairstyles worn by colleagues at your salon. Some styles work better if the hair is not shampooed very often. Other styles need a regular shampoo. Create a simple list of hairstyles which require less frequent shampooing and hairstyles that require more frequent shampooing.

Memory jogger

What is the natural pH of hair?

Why is a steamer used?

What type of water would you use in a steamer?

What massage movements are commonly used when conditioning?

Which massage movements are used mainly when shampooing?

When might you use tepid water to shampoo and condition a client's hair? Why?

Shampooing hair (4)

Massage techniques

During the shampoo and application of conditioner, you will need to use certain massage movements. The most popular movements used within the salon are:

- effleurage
- rotary
- petrissage.

The amount of shampoo you use for each client will be different depending on the length and thickness of their hair. A small amount of shampoo, no bigger than the size of a ten pence piece, is usually sufficient. Dispense the shampoo into the palm of your hand. Rub both palms together and then place the palms of your hands on the client's hair, smoothing the shampoo on to the scalp and down the hair length.

You can now use the massage movements. For a thorough shampoo and conditioning treatment, make sure your massage techniques achieve an even distribution of product over the hair and scalp. Take care not to pull your client's hair or scratch their scalp. This will cause irritation and discomfort to your client and may prevent the next part of the hair service from being carried out.

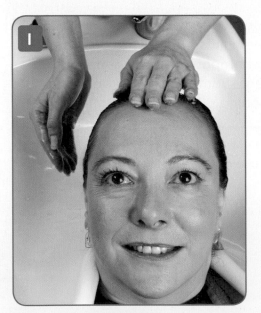

Effleurage movement

Effleurage is used to spread the shampoo throughout the hair at the start of the shampoo and each time you repeat the application of shampoo. Effleurage is a light, slow and superficial movement used as a linking movement to rotary massage.

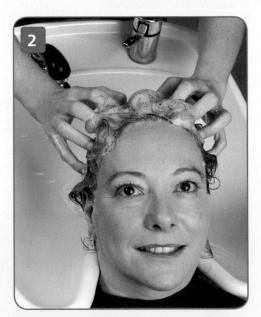

Rotary massage

Rotary massage is used during the shampoo. It is much deeper and faster than effleurage. Your hands should be claw-like when positioned on the client's scalp and should move in small, fast, circular movements with a firm pressure.

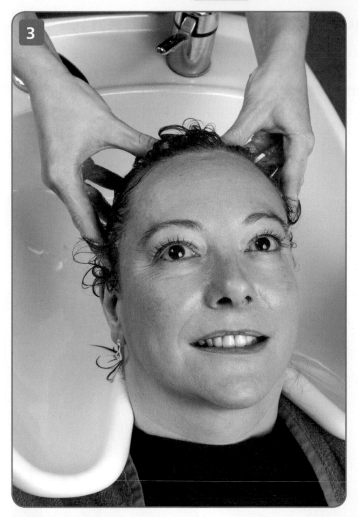

Petrissage movement

Petrissage is a slower version of the rotary movement and is used when carrying out a conditioning treatment. It should totally relax the client, assist penetration of the conditioner and promote blood circulation. Petrissage helps to make the hair smooth, shiny and manageable.

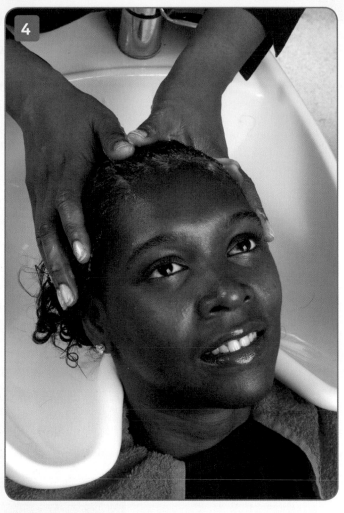

Friction massage

Friction is a massage movement that involves a fast rubbing technique and has a light, gentle plucking action. It is sometimes used when shampooing or when applying lotions such as astringents.

» Get up and go!

Find out from a colleague at your salon what an astringent is and what it is used for.

Applying and removing conditioners (I)

When you have completed the shampoo, you may have to apply conditioning products using the effleurage and petrissage massage movements. Always apply conditioners to the hair following the stylist's and manufacturer's instructions. A conditioning treatment will smooth down the cuticle scales, maintain moisture levels, protect and promote shine and improve the feel of the hair.

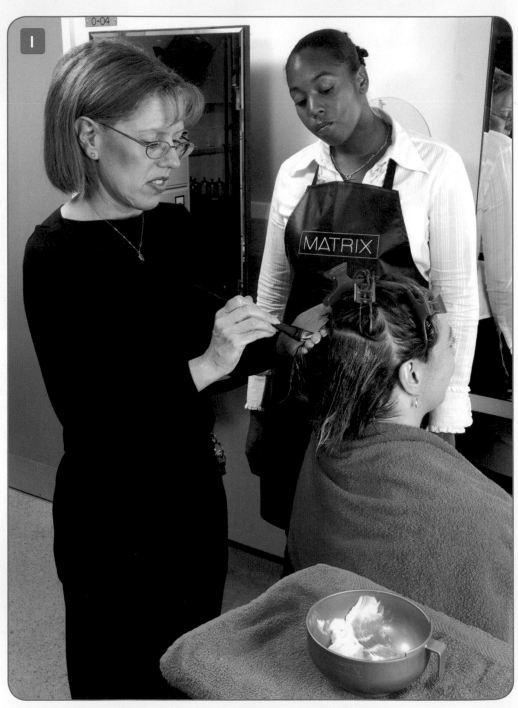

Surface conditioner is applied to protect and promote shine

When removing conditioning products it is important to:

- avoid disturbing the direction of the cuticle
- comb through your client's hair without causing damage to the hair and scalp
- leave your client's hair free of excess water and product.

Should any problems occur, speak promptly to the relevant person in your salon.

After you have finished shampooing and conditioning, rinse the hair thoroughly. This is important to the success of the following treatment. Stylists do not want to ask their client to return to the basin to have excess product removed from the hair. Towel-dry the hair and wrap it in a towel, using a turban style. If you have used a steamer, rinse the client's hair with cooler water than you shampooed with. This will help to smooth down the cuticle scales of the hair ready for styling.

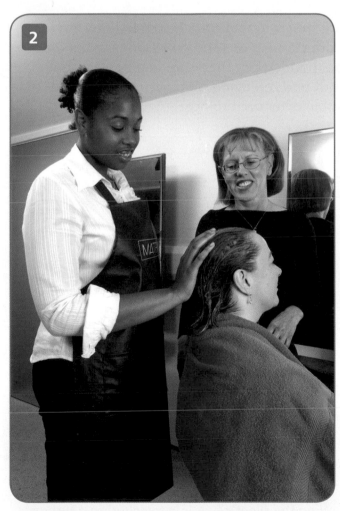

Using effleurage massage when applying conditioner

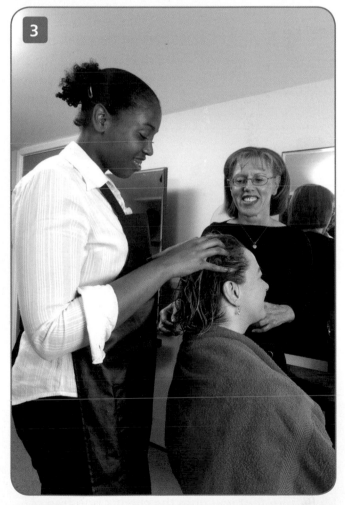

Using petrissage massage when applying conditioner

Applying and removing conditioners (2)

Completing the shampooing and conditioning treatment

The stylist will need you to leave the client's hair free of excess moisture and tangle-free. You will need to comb through from the points to the roots of the hair, without causing any damage to the hair and scalp in preparation for the next treatment.

The client will welcome any advice or guidance you can offer about how to maintain their newly conditioned hair at home. Always be knowledgeable about the products your salon sells. Discuss with your client, at the consultation stage and at the basin, the suitability of professional shampoo and conditioning products. This will help maintain the moisture level of your client's hair and offer protection in between salon visits, particularly if they are having a chemical treatment such as a colour or a perm.

If a client tells you they are shortly going on a beach holiday, advise them to pack hair-care products such as sunscreen, leave-in conditioner and moisturising shampoo. In addition, they can help protect their hair by covering it with a sun hat and removing all traces of chlorine and sea water as soon as possible after swimming.

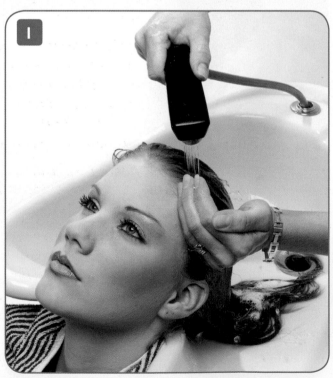

Make sure that you rinse the client's hair free of conditioner

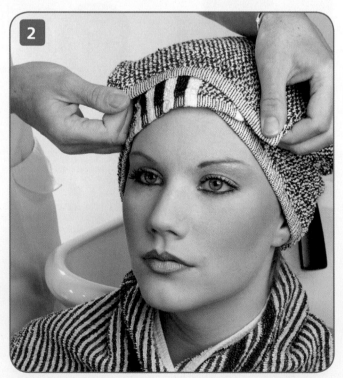

Wrap the client's hair in a towel using a turban style

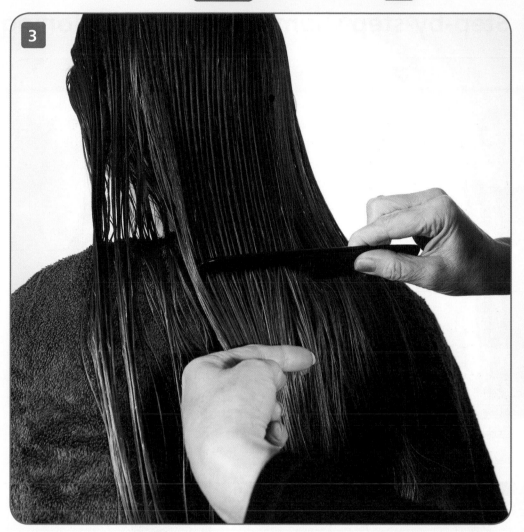

3

Comb through the client's hair, leaving it ready for the next service

Get up and go!

With a colleague, create a list of the physical and chemical treatments an average head of hair may experience, considering how conditioning treatments may be able to help in each case.

Memory jogger

What temperature of water would you choose to rinse off a conditioning treatment?

Why is the flow of water important when shampooing and conditioning?

Why is it important to comb the client's hair from points through to roots following a shampoo and conditioning treatment?

When would you choose not to apply a conditioner?

Why remove excess moisture from the client's hair following the shampoo and condition?

What advice might you give a client going on a beach holiday about looking after their hair?

Get ahead

Now you know how shampoos and conditioners can affect the hair, you might want to learn a little about how water affects hair. Did you know there are two different types of water: hard and soft? Each can affect hairdressing considerably. One can be more damaging than the other, particularly to the electrical equipment that steams or heats the water.

Find out which type of water area you work in and how this type of water can affect hairdressing. If you are in a hard water area, what measures can you take to prevent the build up of limescale? Write up your findings and present them to your colleagues. Can you make it into a mini-teaching session?

Step-by-step shampoo and conditioning

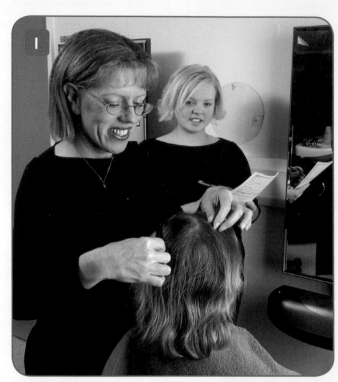

Gown up the client and analyse her hair and scalp before shampooing

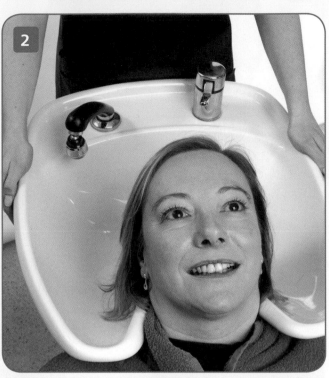

Ensure the client is positioned comfortably before shampooing

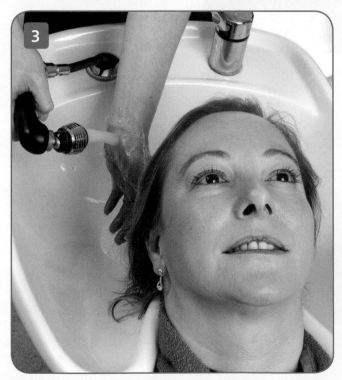

Test the temperature of the water before wetting the client's hair

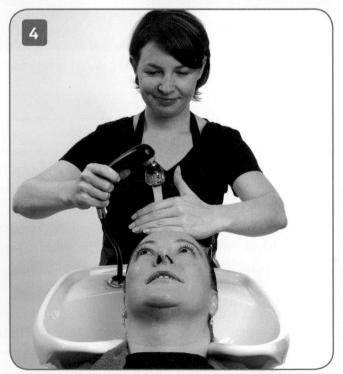

Apply the water to the client's hair, taking care not to wet her face

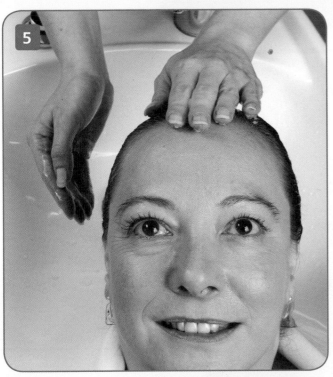

Using effleurage massage, apply the shampoo

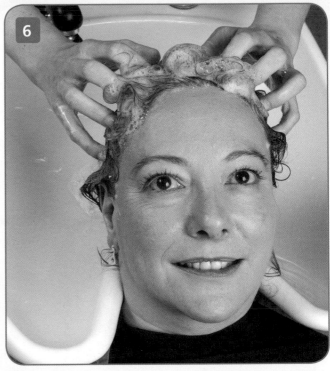

Use rotary massage over the whole head until the shampoo lathers and then rinse the hair free from shampoo

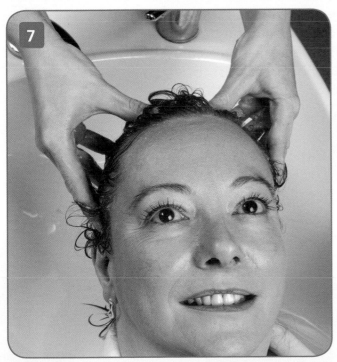

Apply the conditioner using both effleurage and petrissage movements. Rinse the conditioner from the hair and turn off the water. Wrap the client's hair in a towel

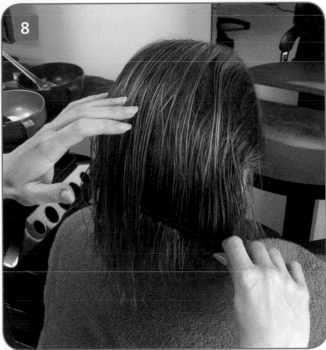

Squeeze the hair to remove excess water. Place a towel around the client's shoulders to prevent any drips and comb through the client's hair ready for further treatment

UNIT GH2

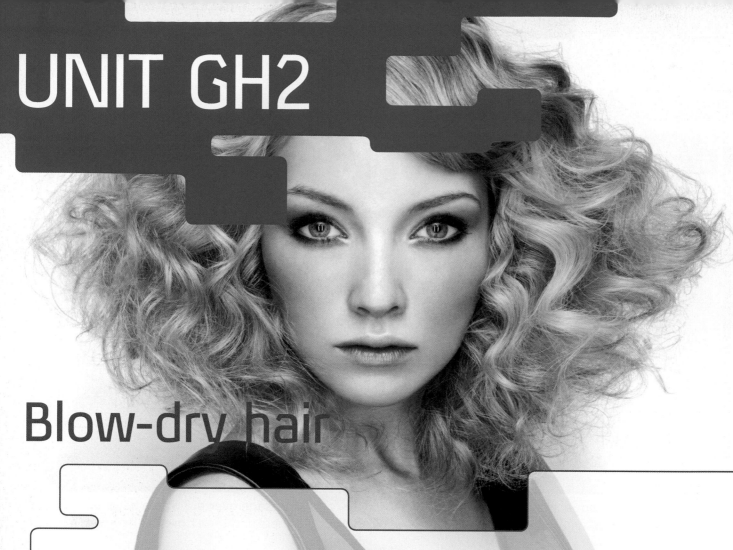

Blow-dry hair

The cut and colour of a hairstyle are of course important, but blow-drying finishes the look. A hairstyle is an expression of a person and their personality – a statement of how they feel. Your client may wear their hair simply and understated at work during the day, but then require a sophisticated or fashionable look for the evening.

A hairstyle needs to complete the overall look the client is after and a professional blow-dry can help them achieve this. It is as important as wearing the right shoes to go with an outfit! Most clients will feel more confident after having a professional blow-dry as part of their treatment, and some will come to your salon for this service alone.

This unit is about carrying out basic blow-drying techniques following the instructions of your stylist, and applies to both hairdressing and barbering salons.

In this unit you will learn how to:

- Maintain effective and safe methods of working when drying hair
- Blow-dry hair.

Here are some key words you will meet in this unit:

Humidity – the amount of moisture in the atmosphere

Cross-infection – an infection that can be passed from one person to another

Infestation – a large number of parasites, e.g. an infestation of the hair and scalp with head lice

Commercially viable time – this basically means good value for money, i.e. hair cut = 30 mins

Disinfection – using chemicals and other methods to reduce the probability of infection

Texture – the way hair feels, determined by touch and helps you decide if hair is porous or non-porous

Cuticle – outside layer of the hair shaft

Cortex – where chemical changes take place in the hair shaft

Medulla – the part of the hair shaft that is full of air spaces and which plays no part when treating hair

Sterilisation – complete destruction of all living organisms

Autoclave – sterilisation system which works under pressure using water

Ultraviolet cabinet – sterilisation system that uses an ultraviolet light to kill bacteria

Maintain effective and safe methods of working when drying hair (I)

Protecting the client

As a first step when working in the salon, you must always protect your client and their clothing when preparing them for their service or treatment. The service could be a non-chemical treatment such as a blow-dry, set, hair cut or conditioning treatment, or perhaps a chemical treatment, such as a colour, bleach or perm. Make sure your client's clothing is effectively protected throughout the service and check with your stylist the most appropriate way to protect them. Many salons use the following items to protect clients:

- **towels**
- **gowns**
- **waterproof capes.**

Of course, all protective equipment should be clean. No one wants to smell the odour of the previous client or a previous treatment on the gown they are wearing. Clean resources also reduce the risk of cross-infection and infestation. Protective equipment should always be in plentiful supply and good condition.

> ## » Get up and go!
>
> Start to buy the *Hairdressers Journal* and use it to put together your own style book. You can then use your style book when you are consulting with clients about how they want their hair to be styled. Remember to consider the different types of clients who may visit your salon and include styles that will appeal to them. Remember to use gents' and children's hairstyles.
>
> Look at your family's and friends' current styles – could you suggest something a little different to complement their features? Think about the practicalities of using your style book. It needs to be durable and waterproof and possibly sectioned into short, medium and long hairstyles.

Positioning your client

You will need to position your client in order to carry out the service, but you should do so without making them uncomfortable. You should also be aware of your own positioning and posture while you are working, ensuring you are minimising the risk of injury to yourself, and others. Having a good posture throughout the working day will help prevent you from feeling physically tired and, as a result, you should be able to work more efficiently.

For the blow-dry service, the client needs to be encouraged to sit square in the chair (not to one side) with their legs uncrossed. Sitting with crossed legs will lead to an unbalanced hairstyle. As the stylist, you need to stand with your feet hip-width apart and distribute your weight evenly over both legs (don't put all your weight onto one leg). Keep your head up and try to avoid stretching over the client or work area. Following these simple steps will minimise the risk of injury and fatigue.

Keeping a safe and clean work area

By keeping your work area clean and tidy throughout the service you will be able to make the best use of your time. If you regularly clear away used resources and things you no longer need, you will be able to access the things you do need easily and without delay. Making effective use of your time also means being organised and planning ahead so you're not constantly going back and forth across the salon to get equipment and products. Remember to prepare items like styling mousse, hairspray and a back mirror for finishing the service. Your client will be impressed at your professionalism and will be happy they are not kept waiting unnecessarily.

To ensure a safe working environment, all tools and equipment must be cleaned and sterilised in the correct way before being used. These measures will minimise the risk of cross-infection and infestation. Use appropriate cleaning materials to clean the areas you are working in and make sure you clean them regularly.

> **? Memory jogger**
>
> What items can be used to protect your clients?
>
> For what reasons should clean protective equipment be used for each new client?
>
> Why should a client be encouraged to sit with their legs uncrossed?
>
> How should you position yourself when working on a seated client?
>
> Why should all tools be cleaned and sterilised prior to each client?
>
> How can you make effective use of your time?

Maintain effective and safe methods of working when drying hair (2)

Sterilisation methods

Moist heat

Moist heat is used in an autoclave, which works rather like a pressure cooker. The distilled water inside the autoclave is heated to a temperature of approximately 125°C and must only be used for small pieces of equipment which have been cleaned using hot soapy water before being put into the autoclave. The autoclave will sterilise hard rubber, such as vulcanized rubber combs, and small metal pieces of equipment such as scissors. This method will make your tools sterile which means they are completely free from all bacteria.

Liquid chemicals (barbicide)

This can be an effective method of sterilising tools, provided the tools have been cleaned with warm soapy water first. The tools must then be immersed in the liquid and left for at least one hour.

Ultraviolet light

An ultraviolet (UV) cabinet uses UV light rays to kill bacteria. Again it is only effective when the tools are cleaned beforehand with warm soapy water. The UV light must reach all surfaces and this means you must turn your equipment in order to sterilise all sides.

Always remember to read and follow the manufacturers' instructions when using your salon's preferred method(s) of sterilisation.

Personal hygiene

As you are working in very close contact with clients and colleagues, you must make sure you smell clean and fresh every day. Personal clothing comes into contact with the skin and must be changed daily. You should also bathe or shower every day to remove body odour. Always use an effective deodorant on clean skin and practise good dental hygiene. Brush your teeth at least twice a day and consider using a mouth freshener such as a mouthwash. Regularly check your breath for stale smells of last night's dinner and perhaps cigarette smoke.

Your hands are in constant use and will carry bacteria from one place to another. Wash them regularly and keep your fingernails clean and free from sharp or broken edges. Cover any cuts in the skin on your hands with a suitable dressing. By having good personal standards of health and hygiene you will be minimising the risk of cross-infection, as well as giving a professional image and not offending your clients!

>> **Get up and go!**

Take photographs in your salon or cut pictures from trade magazines of each of the following pieces of equipment: back mirror, combs, crimpers, flat brushes, handheld dryer, heated rollers, hood dryer, hot brushes, rollers, round brushes, section clips, straighteners, tongs.

Make a collage of the tools and equipment you are likely to work with every day. Perhaps you could involve a few colleagues and develop this as a small project.

? Memory jogger

Name three methods of sterilising tools and equipment in the salon.

What is the most effective method of sterilising small pieces of equipment in the salon?

Before using your chosen method of sterilisation, what must you do to your tools and equipment?

State the common name of one infestation you are most likely to find in a hairdressing salon.

How can you prevent body odour and bad breath?

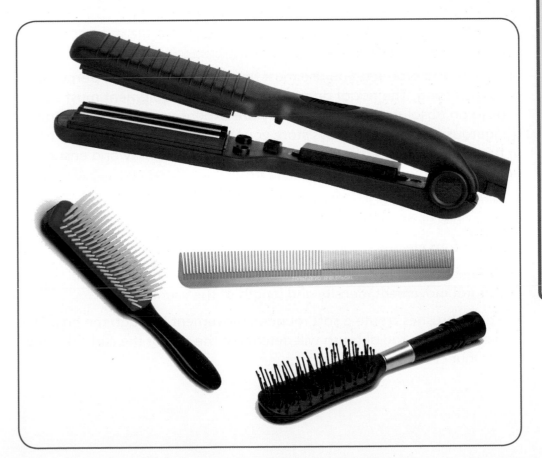

Blow-dry hair (1)

In order to complete this unit successfully, you must carry out blow-dry services on two different hair lengths: above and below the shoulders, creating volume and movement. Pages 114–117 show step-by-step procedures for these.

Before you carry out a blow-dry service, you should always:

- work closely with the stylist and follow their instructions
- ask questions to check you understand
- be sure there is agreement between you, the stylist and the client regarding the desired style
- check what type of products you will be using, if required at all.

If you are unsure or do not understand, always double check with your stylist or a senior member of staff.

Observation

Watch your stylist as part of your professional development and take note of how they control their styling tools and equipment to minimise the risk of damaging the hair or causing the client discomfort. These skills must be practised many times before becoming perfect. The direction of airflow is important to achieving the desired look and avoiding damage to the hair cuticle.

Tools and products

The tools and products you use must be safe and fit for the purpose of hairdressing. The risk of damage to tools and equipment must be kept to an absolute minimum as they are expensive and may be made dangerous as a result. Always store your salon's equipment safely and in the correct place – this will give good value for money and ensure equipment remains in good working order.

- Make sure there are no kinks or knots in the cables of your dryer or other pieces of equipment.

- Never turn electrical equipment on or off with wet hands.

- When choosing brushes to blow-dry with, consider the texture, natural movement, density and length of the client's hair.

- Radial brushes create a soft rounded movement through the hair. The diameter of a radial brush will determine the size of the curl achieved on your client's hair.

- Using straighteners requires a steady hand and careful handling. Straighteners reach very high temperatures in a matter of seconds and you must know how to use them before attempting to use them on clients. They must always be used on dry hair and you should check the client's hair is in good enough condition to cope with the high temperature. For the time being, you may be able to use them on a client only under close supervision. For best results, take small sections, comb through and place the hair between the two plates. Gently close the plates and take the straighteners through the length of hair, allowing the section to drop. This will smooth the cuticle layer of the hair shaft and give a very professional finish to the style.

- Since working in a salon, you have probably noticed the tools of the trade are often personal to the stylist. Many stylists have favourite brushes, combs and scissors and are not always happy to share their equipment. Should you ever need to borrow a piece of equipment, be respectful by looking after it and returning it as soon as possible, clean and sterilised.

» Get up and go!

Draw up a list of the different styles which are achieved through blow-drying in your salon. Consider hair lengths and hair types.

Ask each stylist how long it would take to complete each blow-dry style, including any additional straightening or tonging. Compare these findings with what is considered to be an acceptable commercial timeframe.

Discuss your findings with each of the stylists. Remember, though: it is not a race, and sometimes hair density can play an important part in the length of time it takes to blow-dry a client's hair.

? Memory jogger

Explain why it is important to direct the airflow from a handheld dryer correctly.

What factors influence the choice of style you will create?

What should you think about when choosing a brush?

Why is it important to know how to use straighteners correctly?

List the tools you need to carry out a blow-dry.

Blow-dry hair (2)

The blow-dry service

Once your client's hair has been shampooed, the style discussed and chosen, and any application of products has been agreed by both your client and stylist, you can then start to blow-dry the client's hair.

The client

Your client must always be looked after throughout the service.

- Regularly check they are comfortable.
- Make sure there isn't any water or product running down the client's face.

Technique

- The blow-dry service must be completed within a commercially viable time and this is usually 30–45 minutes, depending on the length, type, density and texture of the client's hair. Make sure your client knows how long the service will take before you start.

- Work on towel-dried hair, not dripping wet hair.

- Don't drop wet hair onto dry hair as this will make the sections you have dried flop and lose shape.

- Wet hair is more delicate than dry. Any tugging may cause hairs to break, as well as causing your client discomfort and annoyance.

- In order to prevent burning your client's skin and hair, causing hair damage or discolouring the hair, keep your dryer moving and always follow the direction of the hair shaft. This will smooth the cuticle layer, giving a sleek, shiny finish.

- When your client's hair is delicate, keep the dryer on a cool setting and at least 1.25 centimetres away from the hair and scalp.

- Show the client the style as you build, develop and work towards the finished look. Use the back mirror and double-check the style is going according to your client's wishes.

- Allow the hair to cool after blow-drying. Doing this fixes the style in place and prolongs the length of time the style will keep its shape. Separate the hair using your fingers or use a tail comb if needed.

- Once you have completed the blow-dry, check with your client and stylist that the style meets both their requirements.

- Apply finishing products such as serum or hairspray if required.

>> Get up and go!

A good hairdresser will always advise their client on ways of maintaining their hairstyle at home. What aftercare advice can you give to your clients? Think about making an 'aftercare card', perhaps the size of a credit card, which you can give to clients after a blow-dry. Make sure the tips are easy to read and keep the information brief. You could include something like:

- Towel dry hair before blow-drying.
- Comb hair from the ends.
- Keep the hairdryer moving all the time.
- Avoid excessive heat.
- Minimise the use of straighteners.
- Remember to protect your hair from the sun.
- Avoid using rubber bands to hold your hair up.
- Use serum on dry hair to protect it.

Get ahead

Look back at the different face shapes on page 4. What styles would you suggest for each?

? Memory jogger

Why should you always advise the client how long a blow-dry will take?

Why should you take care to keep wet hair away from pre-dried hair?

Why should sections of hair be kept damp before blow-drying?

When giving a blow-drying service, when should you show the client their hair in the back mirror?

What are the benefits of allowing hair to cool before dressing out?

Why is it important to give your client aftercare advice?

Blow-dry hair (3)

Blow-drying using a radial brush

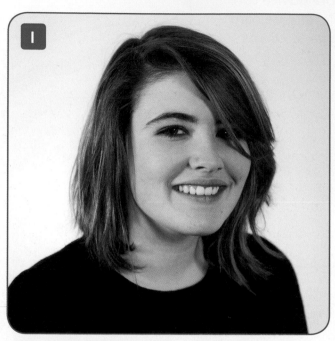

Correctly gown the client and, after your consultation, take them to the basin for shampooing and conditioning

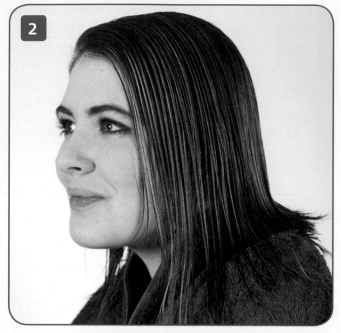

After rinsing, towel dry the client's hair and comb through before you begin to section

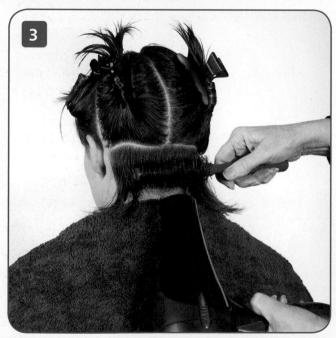

Place the brush horizontally into the section of hair and take through to the ends, wrapping the ends around the brush. Follow through with the dryer and dry from the roots to points

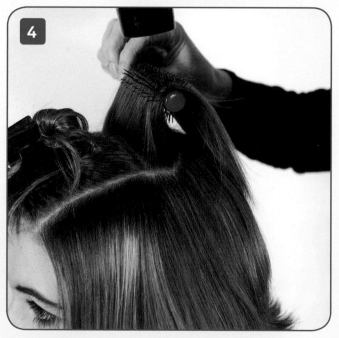

To encourage root lift, lift sections straight up from the crown. Check with your client if the style is developing as required

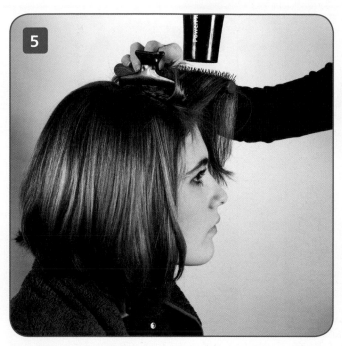

Position yourself parallel to the section you are working on and complete the front section

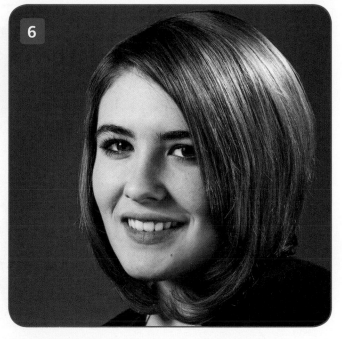

Apply products such as spray or serum to complete the look as required

Blow-dry hair (4)

Blow-drying using a flat-backed brush

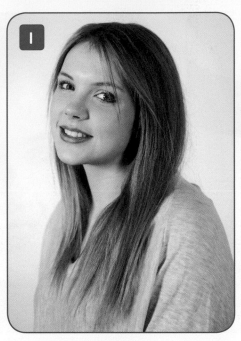

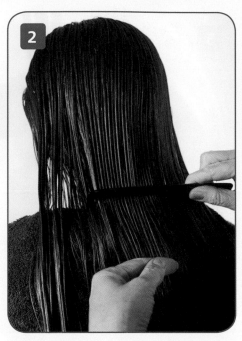

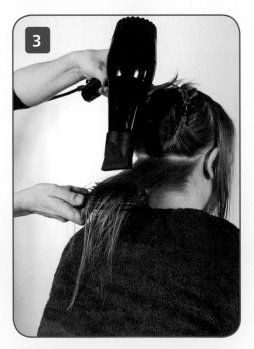

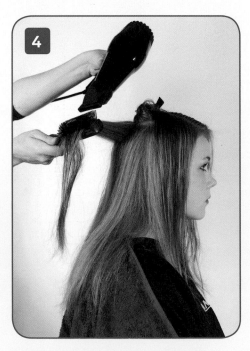

Correctly gown the client and, after your consultation, take them to the basin for shampooing and conditioning

After rinsing, towel dry the client's hair and comb through before you begin to section

Place the flat brush under the roots of the hair and blow dry, encouraging root lift and volume. Keep the dry hair from falling onto wet hair

Continue to move through the blow dry from the nape to the occipital bone, remembering to incorporate the sides of the client's head

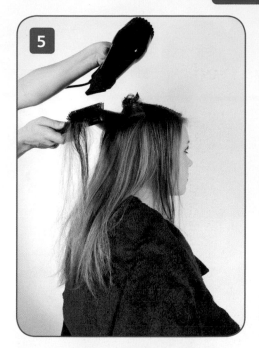

To encourage a smooth and shiny look, direct the dryer down the hairshaft

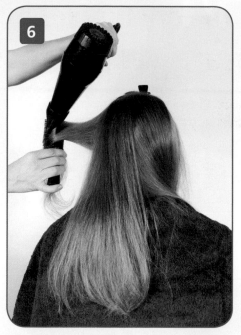

You should stand parallel to the section you are blow drying when incorporating the sides. Check with the client if they are happy with the style as it develops

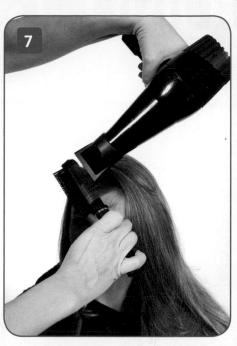

Angle the dryer and brush to finish the fringe area

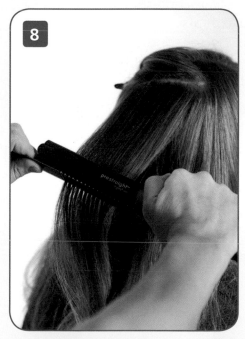

Use straighteners and a comb for a polished finish

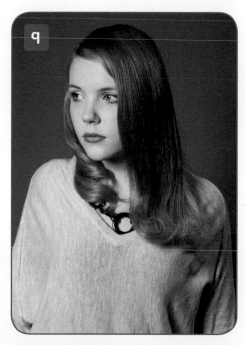

The finished look – apply products such as spray or serum to complete the look as required

UNIT GH4

Assist with hair colouring services

Anne Veck, photographer: Julian Knight

Not everyone is happy with their natural hair colour. Some of your clients may feel that their natural colour doesn't suit them, they have too much grey or that their style may look more up to date with a colour change. With the help of their salon, it is now possible for clients to achieve a natural looking hair colour change – or not so natural, if they want an unusual colour! Colouring hair can also add depth and shine, as well as lift the natural hair colour and leave it in better condition than before. Your clients do not even have to commit to a permanent colour, so can change their mind later and try something completely different.

This unit is about the basic skills of removing colouring and lightening products. The work involved will be carried out under the direction of the relevant person such as the stylist or assessor. This unit will apply for hairdressing students working in hairdressing and barbering salons.

In this unit you will learn about:

- Hair colour
- Maintaining effective and safe methods of working when assisting with colouring services
- Removing colouring and lightening products.

Here are some key words you will meet in this unit:

Dermis – the inner layer of the skin

Pigment – a substance that colours something

Emulsify – using the colouring product to help remove itself by moving the finger pads around the client's hairline

Eumelanin – brown/ black pigment in the hair

Pheomelanin – red/yellow pigment in the hair

Cortex – layer of the hair where chemical changes take place

Cuticle – outer layer of the hair shaft

Surface conditioner – conditioner which coats the outer layer of the hair shaft

Antioxidant conditioner – conditioner which penetrates into the cortex layer of the hair shaft

Tangle-free – hair which has been combed smooth and is free from knots or tugs

Minimise – reduce the effect of something

Fatigued – weary; exhausted from over work or adopting a poor posture

Hair colour

What gives hair its natural colour?

Hair colour is genetic, which means the natural colour of your hair is a result of the mixture of both your mum's and your dad's genes. You do, however, usually receive a predominant gene for hair colour from either your mum or your dad, e.g. your mum/dad might have a strong red pigment as their natural colour. This colour may then dominate your natural colouring.

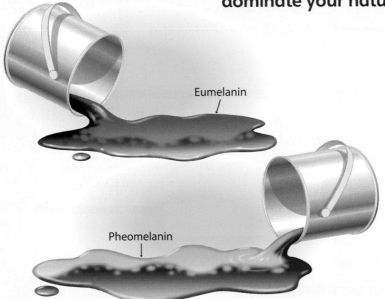

Eumelanin

Pheomelanin

When we look more closely at the process of how hair develops beneath the skin, we can see how hair colour cells produce colour. Cells called melanocytes in the cortex of the hair shaft produce two colour pigments called:

- eumelanin
- pheomelanin.

Everyone has varying proportions of eumelanin and pheomelanin. People who have naturally brown or black hair will have lots of the pigment eumelanin. People who have red or blonde hair will have more of the pigment pheomelanin.

Which pigment have you got more of: eumelanin or pheomelanin?

≫ Get up and go!

Gather together some paints in primary colours (red, yellow and blue). Mix together in equal quantities:

- red and blue
- red and yellow
- yellow and blue.

What new colours did you create? You should have created purple, orange and green. These are secondary colours. By changing the amounts of each primary colour you mix together, you can create your very own colour. Which colours complement each other and go together well? Which ones don't go so well together? Be creative and make decisions about the colours you are making and mixing. Colouring hair can be creative and fun, and you can apply some of the skills you have just learned when in the salon.

Shades of hair colour

Colours come in different shades, which is how light or dark they are. When you look at a hair shade chart you will notice there is a numbering system. Hair shades are numbered between one and ten, with ten being the lightest (blonde) and one being the darkest (black).

Black, brown, red or blonde?

As we have already learned, hair colour comes from the pigments produced in the hair shaft. Different combinations of these pigments produce the many different natural colours and shades of hair. If a person has no pigments in the hair shaft, he or she will have white hair – this is due to the melanocytes no longer producing colour pigment. Reasons for white hair include ageing, heredity, trauma, shock, stress or childbirth. Interestingly, redheads have more hair than brunettes, and brunettes have more hair than blondes.

Colouring hair in the salon

Chemical treatments such as hair colouring and lightening may be offered in your salon. A new hair colour can completely change a client's look. Some of your clients may have experimented with colouring at home, which can be fun and done in no time at all. However, a professional colouring service carried out at a salon can give a much better result, with the added benefit of an expert opinion on what colour to go for.

Your salon may stock the following colouring products:

- temporary colours
- semi-permanent colours
- quasi-colours
- permanent colours
- lightening products
- vegetable colours.

The rest of this unit will deal with working effectively and safely when assisting with colouring services. You will also learn about removing colouring and lightening products from the hair, and materials such as foils, Easi Meche and the highlighting cap.

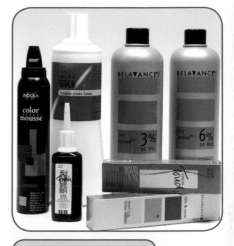

A range of colouring products

? Memory jogger

Name the two pigments found in hair colour. Which gives black/brown hair? Which gives blonde/red hair?

What happens if a hair contains no pigment?

How do hair shade charts work?

» Get up and go!

Test some hair samples with different types of colour. Note down the differences in hair condition and the colour result achieved. Perhaps you can make up your own shade chart.

Maintain effective and safe methods of working when assisting with colouring services (I)

Protecting the client

When preparing a client for a colouring service, or any other service, you must make sure they are properly protected. Use clean towels, gowns and waterproof capes. Follow the instructions of the stylist; they will tell you how best to protect the client, and may ask you to use specific towels for chemical treatments such as colouring.

Don't forget to take care of the client by offering them a drink and a magazine. The best time to do this is probably when the chemical treatment is processing.

Preparing the client for shampooing

Before shampooing, you will need to comb through the client's hair. Remove tangles carefully to avoid causing the client any discomfort. Check the client's scalp with the stylist, looking for any cuts or areas of irritation that may need special attention. You will also need to discuss with the stylist the correct shampoo to use.

> **» Get up and go!**
>
> Does your salon have a towel system? Find out if they do and, if so, what colour towels are used for different treatments. For example, what towel would you use for a permanent colour? What colour towel you would use for a bleach treatment?
>
> Salons use a lot of towels each day. Encourage your salon to go green, if it isn't already. This means washing towels on a cool or warm water programme. The electricity bill will be lower and the salon's energy usage will be more efficient, which is better for the environment.

Personal protective equipment (PPE)

You must always remember to wear personal protective equipment (PPE) when working with clients who are receiving a chemical treatment. Your hands and clothing must be protected at all times. Dermatitis is caused by an irritant coming into contact with the skin and can make skin dry, itchy and sore. Use barrier cream or a good quality hand cream when working in the salon to help prevent your skin from drying out. Protect your skin completely by wearing gloves when applying colouring products, rinsing colours and using hydrogen peroxide or bleaching products.

Positioning the client and checking your own posture

As you are preparing the client for shampooing, ask whether they would prefer a front-wash or backwash basin if a choice is available. Position the client at the basin and make sure they are comfortable. Make sure the client's neck is positioned correctly in the curve of the basin, otherwise the nape area may not be shampooed properly. By thinking about your own posture and standing correctly while shampooing you can reduce the risk of injury and fatigue. It is also a good idea to offer the client a towel to safeguard against unavoidable splashes.

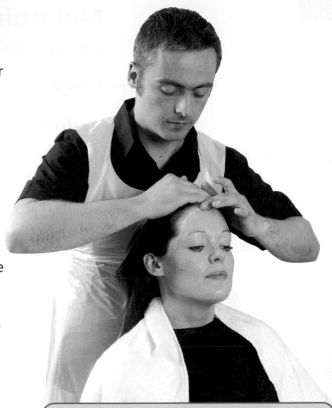

Always wear personal protective equipment when carrying out a chemical treatment

Keeping your work area clean and tidy

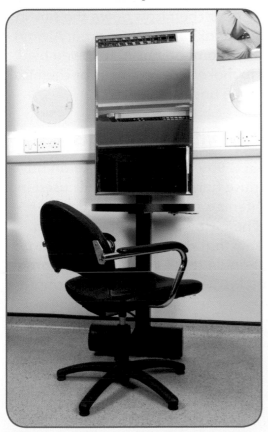

The work area should be kept clean and tidy

It is essential to keep your work area clean and tidy during chemical treatments. Think about the tools, equipment and products you are going to need and make sure you have them to hand. Clear away anything that has been used and won't be needed again. This will ensure you don't waste time or keep your client waiting while you go back and forth getting things, or look for the things you need in a messy work area. Keeping your work area clean and tidy will enable you to work more effectively and it also helps keep your workplace safe.

? Memory jogger

What should always be done before shampooing the client?

What does PPE stand for? Give some examples of PPE, along with when and why they should be used.

What is dermatitis and what causes it? How can you prevent it?

Why might you use a front-wash basin?

How would a dirty and untidy work area affect your work?

Maintain effective and safe methods of working when assisting with colouring services (2)

Reducing product wastage

Before using chemicals, always read the manufacturer's instructions and discuss them with the stylist. If you are asked to mix a chemical product, remember to mix only the amount you need just before it is to be used. Some manufacturers advise using scales to weigh the product, or you may use a measuring beaker instead in order to achieve an accurate mixture. Taking these steps will help to reduce product wastage. If extra product is required, it is more cost-effective to make it freshly as it is needed.

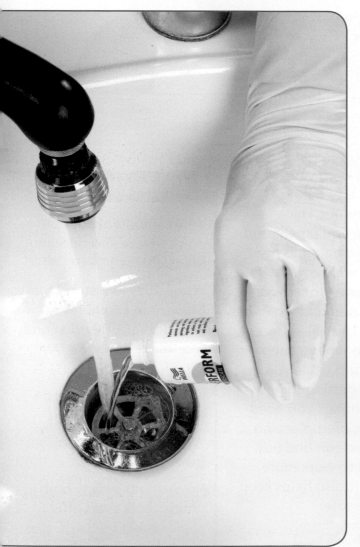

Disposal of chemicals

It is very important that you dispose of chemicals in the proper manner. Your salon must follow the Control of Substances Hazardous to Health (COSHH) Regulations (see page 26) and ensure products are disposed of in a safe and environmentally friendly way. Some salons have a specific basin for disposing of chemicals. Never pour chemicals down the sink in the salon's food and drink preparation area. Always flush them down the shampoo basin, followed by lots of cool water to make sure no smells or chemical waste linger round the basin.

Working safely with chemicals

Some of the products you will use in the salon have the potential to cause harm. The chemicals used in colouring and lightening treatments can damage clothing, skin and hair. However, if they are used correctly it is unlikely that anything will go wrong. You must always handle these chemicals with great care and follow all instructions given to you about their use.

> Chemical waste should be flushed down the shampoo basin

You can reduce the amount of contact a chemical has with the client's skin by using barrier cream around the hairline. You should also always check you are using the right type of heat with each product or you could cause the client to suffer from chemical burns. If you ever have any concerns or problems, it is best to check with the stylist or assessor promptly and find out the correct course of action to take.

Re-ordering products

If the stock levels of a product are running low, remember to follow your salon's policy for re-ordering, which will probably involve telling the appropriate member of staff or writing it down. This will ensure you have sufficient products available, and also avoid having too much stock.

>> **Get up and go!**

With a colleague, find out:

- the different types of colouring and lightening products available in your salon
- how they are applied
- how long they last on the hair.

Reducing the risk of harm or injury to yourself, your colleagues and clients

Always keep a look out for hazards or risks which may arise during the course of the day. Clear away used product bottles and used materials such as bowls and cotton wool. Keep the floor clear from trailing cables, towels, gowns and cut hair, as well as items belonging to clients such as handbags, shopping bags, walking sticks and pushchairs. This will help to minimise the risk of any accidents occurring.

? Memory jogger

Why wouldn't you mix up all the chemicals you need for the day's appointments at the start of the day?

What might happen as a result of pouring chemicals down the basin used for washing up and preparing drinks?

How would you use barrier cream to protect your client?

How can you reduce the risks of accidents in your salon?

Maintain effective and safe methods of working when assisting with colouring services (3)

Reducing the risk of cross-infection

Cross-infection is when an infection is passed from one person to another. You can take some very simple steps as you work to reduce the risk of this happening. Remember to always practise good personal hygiene and wear clean, well-pressed clothes. If you or any of your clients are showing signs of infection or infestation, you must report it straight away to a senior member of staff. They can then advise you what to do. You should also make sure you know how to use your salon's methods of sterilisation properly and ensure you always use clean tools and equipment on each new client.

It is not just for reasons of hygiene that tools and equipment should be properly cleaned. Cleanliness can also make the difference between achieving a professional result and a poor result from colouring and lightening. Make sure brushes and mixing bowls are always washed free of product so as not to contaminate the next product they will be used with. You should also have a different brush for each product you are applying. For example, do not mix bleach with a tint brush that has been used for applying a raspberry grape tint!

 Sharpen up!

In error, you use a tint brush for bleaching which was used previously to apply a rich red colour, but had not been washed out properly. What would happen to the client's hair colour?

Skin tests

Client preparation for colouring and lightening treatments varies from salon to salon, but it is very likely a skin test will need to be carried out 24–48 hours before the service can take place. This will ensure it is safe for the treatment to go ahead and the client won't suffer from any reaction to the product when it is applied. Skin tests will almost certainly be required for most semi-permanent colours, quasi-colours and permanent colours, but may also be needed for vegetable colours too. You must follow the instructions you are given for skin tests very carefully or the consequences could be serious. The results must be recorded on the client's record card.

If your client has sensitive skin or has reacted to other products, natural products such as vegetable colours can sometimes be safer alternatives. They are unlikely to cause dermatitis and do not usually require a skin test. Remember, though, not all clients can use natural products on their skin, so it is still worth checking the suitability first. The processing of vegetable colours may require exposure to oxygen in the atmosphere, which means the final colour result will not be achieved until the day after the treatment.

Incompatibility tests

Another type of test that may be carried out is an incompatibility test. This is where the stylist makes sure the client's hair is able to be coloured or lightened. Previous treatments or hair in poor condition can cause undesirable results. For example, metallic salts which are found in hair colour restorers and compound henna may cause the hair to boil, bubble and break during lightening treatments. If metallic salts are suspected, the stylist will not proceed. As with skin tests, the results should always be noted on the client's record card.

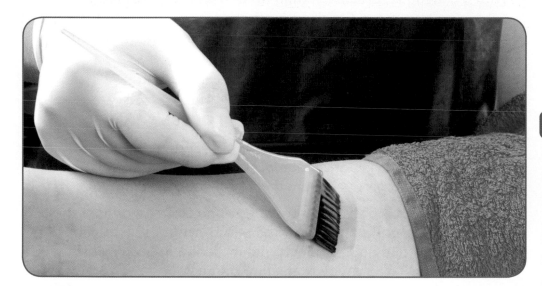

Carrying out a skin test

Get up and go!

With the help of a stylist, carry out an incompatibility test. You will need:

- a sample of hair
- a non-metallic bowl
- hydrogen peroxide
- perm lotion.

Ask your stylist about other types of hair and scalp tests, such as porosity tests and elasticity tests.

? Memory jogger

What can you do to reduce the risk of cross-infection?

How soon before a colouring or lightening treatment should a skin test be carried out?

Are vegetable colours always safe to use on everyone?

Why is an incompatibility test carried out?

Where should the results of any test be recorded?

Removing colouring and lightening products (I)

Resources for colouring and lightening

You will need to prepare a trolley for the stylist with the following items:

- client record card
- clean towels (of the appropriate colours)
- barrier cream
- cotton wool
- shade chart
- foils or Easi Meche
- highlighting cap and hook
- tinting bowl and brush
- hydrogen peroxide (sometimes).

>> **Get up and go!**

With a colleague, practise setting up a trolley for a colour or lightening treatment. Check each other's trolleys for any missing items. Now set up a trolley for each other, but deliberately forget one item. See if you can spot what is missing.

Assisting with the colouring process

Your role in the colouring process includes preparing the client for the treatment and removing any materials (such as foils, a highlighting cap or Easi Meche) and products from the hair after the treatment.

Always check with the stylist before removing colouring or lightening products and materials and follow the manufacturer's instructions. You must learn to remove products and materials in a way which minimises the risk of damage to the hair and colour being spread to the client's skin, clothing and surrounding areas of hair. Some colouring and lightening products require you to emulsify them before water is applied to the hair and scalp. This is important as the colour will not come off the skin if you miss this simple step.

Should there be any problems, refer them to the relevant person, usually the stylist, who will advise you what to do. The types of problems you may come across include the following.

- Colour bleeding onto an area of hair that has not been coloured.
- Bleach splashing into a client's eyes.
- Ripped hair, caused by the highlighting cap being removed roughly.
- An unsatisfactory result, which can be caused by Easi Meche or foils being removed before the end of the processing time.

The table below shows some common colouring problems and how to deal with them.

Fault	By whom	Correction	How to avoid
Colour seepage	Stylist	Recolour areas as necessary	Apply barrier cream to the areas not being coloured
Bleach in client's eyes	Stylist	Rinse with cool water immediately	Careful removal of colouring materials and products
Vigorous removal of the highlighting cap	Junior	Condition hair and massage scalp	Apply conditioner to the top of the cap before removing
Hair colour too warm	Stylist	Apply toner	Check base shade and use correct strength of products

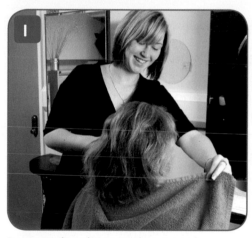

Protect the client with a towel, gown and waterproof cape

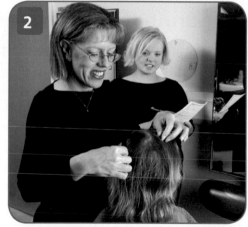

Prepare the client for colouring with the stylist. This involves hair and scalp analysis, and combing and sectioning dry hair

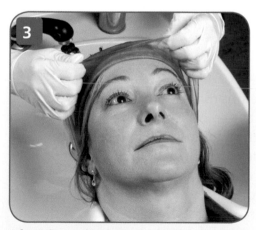

After the stylist has applied the colour and it has been allowed to process, remove the colouring products

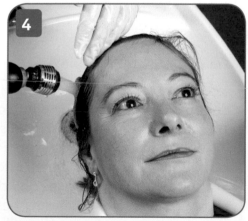

Rinse the hair

Removing colouring and lightening products (2)

Applying conditioner

Once you have removed all of the colouring or lightening product, you may have to use a colour removal shampoo. Following this, squeeze out excess moisture from the hair then apply a suitable antioxidant conditioner or surface conditioner. Antioxidant conditioners will need to be left on the hair for at least three minutes. Antioxidant conditioners will:

- replace lost moisture
- help prevent further oxidation of the hair
- return the pH of the hair to its normal acid value.

Ask your stylist which conditioner to use.

Preparing the client for the next treatment

After rinsing the conditioner from the client's hair, towel-dry the hair and scalp and make sure they are free from excess products and moisture. Help the client to the styling area and comb the hair through, leaving it tangle-free without damaging the hair or scalp. Both the stylist and client need to be satisfied that you have removed all traces of product from the client's hair. Should you have any concerns about the products or how to use them, promptly refer any problems to your stylist or assessor for the appropriate course of action.

Remember to clean and tidy the basin area after you have prepared the client for the next treatment. Make sure all used products are disposed of correctly and leave the area free from risks of hazard, cross-infection or infestation, ready to be used by the next client.

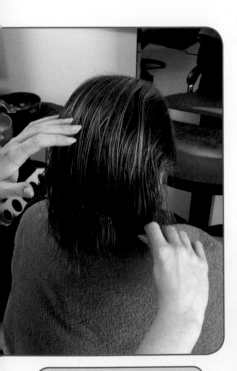

Comb through the client's hair leaving it ready for further treatment

✂ Sharpen up!

You could try to interest clients in temporary colours by wearing a suitable colour in your own hair at the salon. Try different coloured hair mascaras, sprays, mousses, setting lotions, glitters and gels. This will allow clients to see how they look and you can then talk about how you applied them and how you shampoo them out. Talk about the advantages and disadvantages of doing this with a senior stylist or your manager before you go ahead. If you can do this, remember not everyone will want pink highlights!

After-colour care

It is important to explain to clients how they should look after their hair at home. After-colour care involves helping the client to maintain the colour of his or her hair at home using the most appropriate shampoo and conditioner for colour-treated hair. This is part of professional client care, and by selling the client the correct products, you will be giving him or her expert advice and guidance which completes the colouring treatment.

⟫ Get up and go!

Find out how to prepare a bleaching product your salon uses by reading the manufacturer's instructions. Discuss the result, and how you found following the instructions, with a senior colleague.

Get ahead

This book contains a number of step by steps, which show how some practical hairdressing tasks are carried out (see page 129 for an example). Have a go at creating your own step by step showing how to apply semi-permanent colour. Take photographs in your salon and then arrange the photos in order so someone could follow the process. You might want to use the following steps as a guide to taking your photos.

- Step 1: The equipment you will need.
- Step 2: Shampooing the client.
- Step 3: Sectioning the hair into four.
- Step 4: Applying the product to the back of the head using either a tint brush and bowl or applicator bottle.
- Step 5: Applying the product to the side of the head.
- Step 6: Applying the product to the top of the head.
- Step 7: Working the product into the hair shaft.
- Step 8: Leaving the colour to process as per the manufacturer's instructions.
- Step 9: Shampooing and rinsing the product off.
- Step 10: The finished dried and styled result.

Perhaps you could display your step by step photos in your salon to help your junior colleagues. You could even create step by steps for other treatments.

? Memory jogger

Colour has run into your client's eyes. What course of action would you take?

Name three things antioxidant conditioner does.

What are the benefits of offering clients aftercare?

UNIT GH5

Assist with perming hair services

The reason some people have straight hair and others have curly hair is down to the shape of the hair shaft. A naturally straight hair has a circular cross-section, whilst a naturally curly hair has an oval cross-section. It is now understood that the hair follicle also has a big part to play in determining the curliness of hair as it affects the shape of the hair shaft, as well as the angle it grows at. In order to make straight hair curly, as happens during a perm, hairdressers have to change the structure of the hair using chemicals. This is now a safe process and can achieve incredible results.

The work involved in this unit should be carried out under the direction of the relevant person, such as the stylist or assessor. This unit will apply to hairdressing students working in both hairdressing and barbering salons, and is suitable for those working with Caucasian and Asian hair types.

In this unit you will learn about:

- What perming is
- Maintaining effective and safe methods of working when assisting with perming services
- Neutralising hair as part of the perming process.

Here are some key words you will meet in this unit:

Cortex – layer of the hair where chemical changes take place

Cuticle – outer layer of the hair shaft

Disulphide bonds – keratin bonds which are linked together in the cortex

Surface conditioner – conditioner which coats the outer layer of the hair shaft

Anit-Oxy conditioner – conditioner which penetrates into the cortex layer of the hair shaft

Tangle-free – hair which has been combed smooth and is free from knots or tugs

Texture – the way hair feels, determined by touch during the consultation

Fatigue – weary; exhausted from over work or adopting a poor posture

Perming – curling hair by using a chemical product

Neutralising – the process that fixes hair into its new shape

Asian hair – the hair shaft is round in shape, straight and/or coarse

Caucasian hair – the hair shaft is oval in shape and can be straight, wavy or curly

What is perming?

The desire to have curly hair is an old one and throughout history women, in particular, have tried various methods to transform their limp, straight hair into a bouncing head of curls. Hair can be made curly by simply wetting it and winding it, as well as through the use of heated styling equipment. These results are only temporary though and often don't achieve the desired look. With a permanent wave (or perm) curls can be chemically added to straight hair, although straight hair will grow back from the roots.

>> **Get up and go!**

List the different ways in which curls or waves can be added to hair without the use of a perm. Discuss these with your stylist, considering the pros and cons of each.

Perms work by using chemicals to cause a permanent change in the structure of keratin, the protein found in hair. There are two main stages to perming hair.

- Stage I: A chemical is added to the hair that breaks open the disulphide bonds, which give hair its elasticity, in the cortex layer of the hair. This stage must be carefully timed to ensure the correct amount of bonds are broken.

The two stages of perming

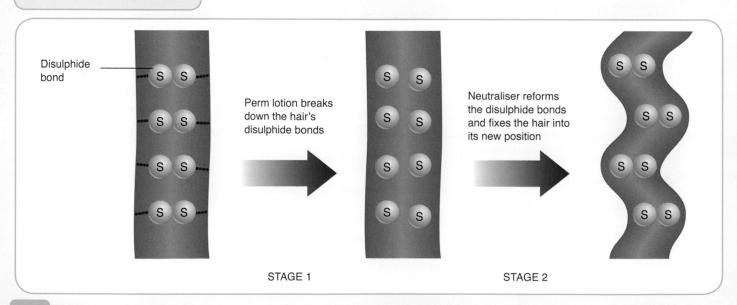

Disulphide bond

Perm lotion breaks down the hair's disulphide bonds

Neutraliser reforms the disulphide bonds and fixes the hair into its new position

STAGE 1   STAGE 2

- Stage 2: A second chemical containing hydrogen peroxide or sodium bromate is used to close the bonds, which causes the hair to take on the shape of the rods. This is called neutralising. Again, timing is essential when completing this stage in order to achieve the desired result and not damage the hair.

Because the change caused by perming is permanent, it can only be removed by cutting or growing the hair out, or reversing the treatment chemically.

Acid and alkaline perms

Perms can be of the acid or alkaline variety. Alkaline perms contain ammonia and have a pH of between 8.2 and 9.6. Acid perms have a pH of between 4.5 and 6.5 (remember, hair is acidic with a pH of between 4.5 and 5.5). Alkaline perms work more quickly than acid perms and usually hold their shape for longer. Acid perms act more slowly and are gentler on the hair. A stylist will choose either an acid or alkaline perm depending on the result required and the client's hair type and condition. Hair which is dry, damaged or porous will be better suited to an acid perm, which is less likely to cause damage.

Considering hair types when perming

Chemical treatments for Caucasian and Asian hair types are slightly different and you will need to be able to work with both. The differences between Caucasian/European and Asian/Oriental hair are important when choosing the most appropriate product. The Caucasian/European hair shaft can be straight, wavy or curly and has an oval cross-section. The Asian hair shaft can be straight and/or coarse and is round in shape.

The texture of hair will vary from client to client and may also vary within the same head of hair. Texture can be fine, medium or coarse, with fine hair having a small circumference and coarse hair a large circumference. To determine the texture, run your fingers along the length of a single hair. This information will be useful when you are choosing products.

> **» Get up and go!**
>
> What types of perm lotion are used in your salon for different hair types and conditions? Discuss them with your senior stylist.

> **? Memory jogger**
>
> Describe the two stages in perming hair.
>
> Why might an acid perm be more suitable for some clients' hair?
>
> Explain the difference between Caucasian/European hair and Asian/Oriental hair.
>
> How can you determine the texture of hair?

Maintain effective and safe methods of working when assisting with perming services (I)

Protecting the client

Make sure your client is suitably protected for the perming service. Use clean gowns, towels and waterproof capes. Your salon may use specific towels for chemical treatments and different ones for non-chemical treatments.

Personal protective equipment (PPE)

Remember to wear personal protective equipment (PPE) when working with clients who are receiving a chemical treatment. Your hands and clothing must be protected at all times. Wear gloves when rinsing perm lotion and neutralising products from the hair. This is to protect yourself from the damage that perming chemicals can potentially cause.

Preparing the client for shampooing

Before shampooing, you will need to comb through the client's hair. Remove tangles carefully to avoid causing the client any discomfort and check the client's scalp with the stylist for any cuts or irritated areas. You will also need to discuss with the stylist the correct shampoo to use.

The pre-perm shampoo

The pre-perm shampoo will remove any build-up of hair-care products, open the cuticles and leave the hair at a neutral pH of 7 ready for either an acid or alkaline perm lotion.

Positioning the client and checking your own posture

Ask the client if they would prefer a backwash or a front-wash basin if available and position them carefully, checking they are comfortable. Remember to think about your own posture during the shampoo so as to reduce the risk of injury or fatigue.

Preparing the resources for perming

You will need to prepare a trolley for the stylist with the following items:

- client record card
- clean towels (of the appropriate colours)
- barrier cream
- cotton wool
- gloves
- apron
- a selection of combs
- a plastic bowl
- plastic cap*
- rods

Sharpen up!

Why might a salon use different coloured towels for perming and neutralising?

- end papers
- section clips
- tension strips
- Climazone or other heat source*

- gown
- waterproof cape.

* These items may be needed

All resources must be cleaned or sterilised after every use. This will help to minimise the risk of cross-infection.

Familiarising yourself with manufacturers' instructions

Here is a typical list of manufacturer's perming instructions.

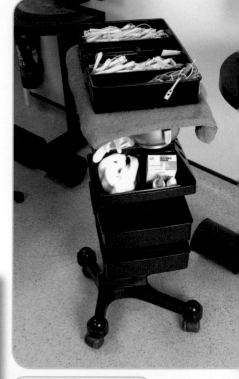

A trolley prepared for perming

Vitality

Vita Perm

Permanent wave

Instructions for use (read thoroughly).

1 Preparation:
- Check the condition and porosity of the hair then select the correct lotion.
- Shampoo the hair using a mild shampoo. Rinse thoroughly and towel-dry.
- To equalise hair porosity for an even curl result, a pre-perm treatment is recommended.
- Section the hair and select appropriate curler size for the chosen technique, then wind without lotion. Vitality End Papers make winding easier.

2 Application:
- Wear protective gloves.
- Carefully apply the perm lotion onto each curler, using the applicator nozzle.
- Repeat if necessary to ensure thorough penetration, but do not over-saturate.
- Allow to develop.

3 Development guidelines:
The suggested development times in the guidelines overleaf have been tested thoroughly and produce optimum results. However, if you are unsure about the overall condition and porosity of the hair, we recommend test curls should be taken to determine the final development time. Development times can be increased as required but care should be taken to avoid over-processing. When correct curl strength is achieved, rinse hair thoroughly for five minutes.

4 Rinsing and neutralising:
After completion of development time rinse all curlers thoroughly (2–3 minutes). Thoroughly blot the curlers to remove excess moisture.

Foam neutraliser:

- Pour 50ml of the neutraliser into a non-metallic bowl.
- Add an equal amount of warm water. The neutraliser is now ready to use.
- For maximum neutralisation, use a neutraliser sponge and apply two thirds of the neutraliser evenly to all the curlers, foam up thoroughly (do not foam up in the bowl).
- Leave to develop for five minutes.
- Gently unwind all the curlers and apply the remaining one third of the neutraliser through the hair.
- Distribute evenly and allow to develop for a further five minutes.
- Rinse thoroughly.
- Blot out excess moisture with a clean towel.

5 After care:
After rinsing out we recommend the use of a suitable after-care treatment.

Vitality UK Ltd. Newtown NW1 1AB

? Memory jogger

Why is it important to wear the correct PPE when assisting with perming services?

Name the three reasons why pre-perm shampoo is used.

List as many of the resources needed for perming as you can.

137

Maintain effective and safe methods of working when assisting with perming services (2)

Assisting with the perming service

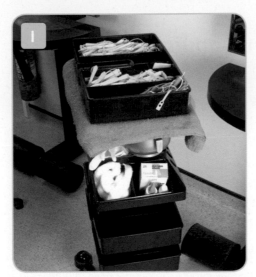

Ensure the trolley is prepared prior to perming

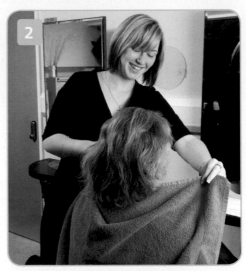

Protect the client with towels, a gown and a cape

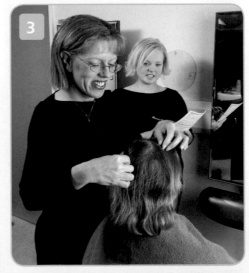

Carry out a hair, skin and scalp analysis by dividing the hair into sections

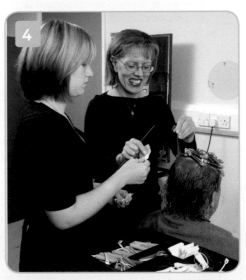

Pass rods and papers to the stylist as they need them

≫ Get up and go!

You could try to interest clients in perming services by wearing your own hair curly. Try curling your hair a couple of times during the week and take notice of the comments your clients make. Talk to them about the advantages of curling their hair and show them suitable styles.

Keeping your work area clean and tidy

Look at page 123 in Unit GH4 to find out how you can keep your work area clean and tidy, and why this is important.

Reducing product wastage

Look at page 124 in Unit GH4 to find out how you can limit the amount of products your salon wastes.

>> Get up and go!

Find out how to prepare a neutraliser your salon uses by reading the manufacturer's instructions. Discuss the result, and how you found following the instructions, with a senior colleague.

>> Get up and go!

With a colleague, find out:

- the different types of perming products available in your salon
- how they are applied
- how long they last on the hair.

Disposal of chemicals

Look at page 124 in Unit GH4 to find out how to properly dispose of chemicals in the salon.

Reducing the risk of harm or injury to yourself, your colleagues and clients

Look at page 125 in Unit GH4 to find out how you can reduce the risk of harm or injury to yourself, your colleagues and clients.

Reducing the risk of cross-infection

Look at page 126 in Unit GH4 to find out what cross-infection is and how you can take some simple measures to reduce the risk of it happening.

? Memory jogger

How would a dirty and untidy work area affect your work?

Why wouldn't you mix up all the chemicals you need for the day's appointments at the start of the day?

How can you reduce the risks of accidents in your salon?

What might happen as a result of pouring chemicals down the basin used for washing up and preparing drinks?

What can you do to reduce the risk of cross-infection?

Where should the results of any test be recorded?

Skin and incompatibility tests

Skin tests involve applying a small amount of a product to the client's skin in order to ensure it is safe for a chemical treatment such as perming to go ahead. The test usually needs to be carried out 24–48 hours before the service can take place. You must follow the instructions you are given for skin tests very carefully or the consequences could be serious.

An incompatibility test involves taking a sample of the client's hair and applying the product to it. This is to make sure the client's hair is in a suitable condition to cope with the chemical treatment. The result of any test must be recorded on the client's record card.

>> Get up and go!

Ask your stylist about other types of hair and scalp tests that are carried out, such as pre-perm test curl, development tests, porosity tests and elasticity tests.

Neutralising hair as part of the perming process (1)

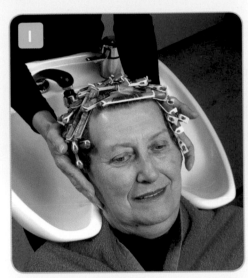

Position the client at the basin and rinse hair thoroughly

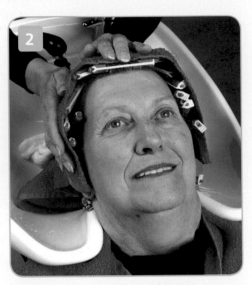

Towel-blot the hair to remove excess water

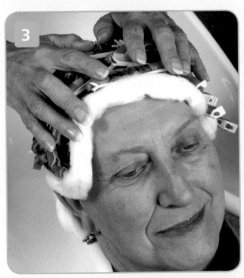

Check there is no excess water by pressing your hands over the rods

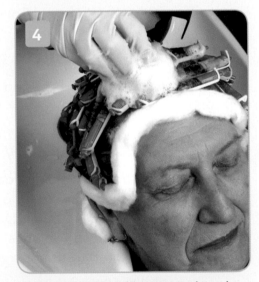

Apply the neutraliser to each rod and allow it to process according to the manufacturer's instructions

>> **Get up and go!**

Discuss with your assessor the reasons why you would not massage or rub the scalp vigorously when rinsing out chemical products.

Rinsing out the perm lotion

You will need to follow both the stylist's and the manufacturer's instructions when rinsing the client's hair free of perm lotion. At the end of the processing time, the hair should be rinsed for a minimum of five minutes to thoroughly remove all traces of perm lotion. It is best to use warm water, which will leave the cuticles of the hair open, enabling the neutraliser to penetrate more effectively.

Towel-blotting the hair

The hair must be free from excess water before the neutraliser is applied. To remove excess moisture, you will need to towel-blot the hair. It is worth taking time to do this properly as too much water in the hair will dilute the neutraliser and ruin the perm. Check how wet the hair is by placing your hands over the rods – if you find lots of water on your hands, you must continue with towel-blotting. Some salons may use tissue or cotton wool to remove excess water from the client's hair.

Applying the neutraliser

As you have already learned, neutraliser closes the bonds that were broken by the perming lotion and fixes the hair into the shape of the rod being used. There are two main types of neutraliser used in the salon:

- hydrogen peroxide neutralisers
- sodium bromate neutralisers.

Correct timing of the neutralising process is crucial to the finished result. Over-processing can leave the hair frizzy, and under-processing will give a weak curl result. Make sure the client's skin is well protected before applying the neutraliser. Use barrier cream and damp cotton wool around the hairline.

You must match the neutraliser with the perm lotion being used. For example, an alkaline perm must be followed through with a hydrogen peroxide neutraliser. Some neutralising products can be used straight from the bottle, whilst others will need foaming up in a bowl first. The stylist will instruct you on how to use a particular product. You should also read the manufacturer's instructions, which will explain how to use the neutraliser safely and effectively.

Make sure you apply the neutraliser evenly throughout the client's wound hair, taking care to avoid any area which has not been permed. Unpermed hair can be protected by applying gel or conditioner. Leave the neutraliser on the client's hair for the recommended length of time. This will ensure the disulphide bonds are fixed into their new position. You may find it helpful to use a timer to accurately time the processing. Some types and lengths of hair may need a longer time to develop depending on the amount of hair wound around the rod.

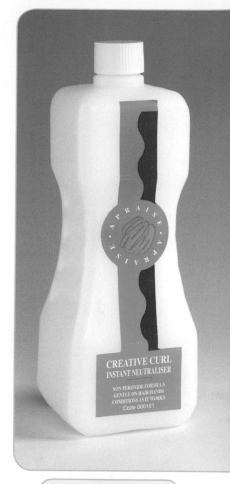

An example of a neutralising product

? Memory jogger

How long do you rinse the client's hair prior to applying neutraliser?

Why towel-blot the hair before applying neutraliser?

Name the two types of neutraliser.

Why is timing the neutralising process correctly so important?

Neutralising hair as part of the perming process (2)

Removing the rods

With some neutralisers you will need to leave the rods in place during processing. Others require you to remove the rods after five minutes before continuing with the second part of the process. Always check the instructions to make sure you are using the product correctly. When you do remove the rods, you will have to do so very carefully so as not to disturb the curl and cause the hair to become straight. The hair is also in a very delicate state at this time and any rough handling can cause irritation to the client's scalp. Check with your stylist whether or not you should apply more neutraliser.

Removing the neutraliser

After the neutraliser has been left to process for the appropriate time, rinse it off thoroughly so that no traces are left in the hair. This will prevent chemical damage to the hair and makes sure the new shape is fixed.

Applying conditioner

Remove excess moisture from the client's hair by squeezing out the water by hand. Then apply a suitable antioxidant conditioner to the client's hair. Leave the conditioner on the hair for at least three minutes and then remove it, rinsing thoroughly. Towel-dry the client's hair and wrap it in a turban style before showing the client to the styling area. Comb through the hair, leaving it tangle-free for the next treatment. Make sure you leave the basin area clean and tidy ready for the next client.

Perming and neutralising problems

Perming and neutralising problems might include the hair returning to its natural straight look if the neutraliser is left in too long, frizziness, uneven curls along the hair length, straight hair at the sides or nape, or an irritable scalp. Mistakes can and do happen in the salon. When they do, stay calm and refer to the senior stylist immediately. To minimise the risk of a problem occurring, make sure you listen to all instructions given to you and check the manufacturer's instructions for each product.

The table opposite shows some common perming problems and how to deal with them.

Fault	By whom	Correction	How to avoid
Fish hooks	Stylist	Remove by cutting	Cover points of hair with end papers
Over-processing	Stylist/Junior	Cut and condition	Carefully time the process using the salon clock or a timer. Record the processing time on the record card
Neutraliser applied unevenly	Stylist/Junior	Re-perm if the condition of hair allows	Check the stylist's/manufacturer's instructions. Monitor application of neutraliser
Skin and scalp irritation	Junior	Rinse immediately with cool water	Carry out appropriate test before chemical treatment
Hair breakage	Stylist	Cut to disguise and use restructurant to strengthen hair	Carry out incompatibility test and pre-perm treatment

»» Get up and go!

Not all product manufacturers produce a post-perm treatment. Some offer a product which can be used across a range of perms. Find out what products you can safely use for which perms. Discuss this with your assessor.

After-perm care

It is important to explain to clients how they should look after their hair at home. After-perm care involves helping the client to maintain their perm at home using the most appropriate shampoo, conditioner and styling products for permed hair. This is part of professional client care, and by selling the client the correct products, you will be giving him or her expert advice and guidance which completes the perming treatment.

Get ahead ⬆

Working either with a colleague or a training head, practise winding a spiral perm. This method of perming is time-consuming and needs you to be confident during the winding process as the sections of hair must be evenly wound around the bendy spiral rod. The hair you work on should be medium to long, towel-dried and in neat workable sections secured with butterfly clips. Start by taking sections of hair from the nape area, working from left to right on section one, alternating each section as you work up the client's head. This method of winding will give a degree of width on one-length hair cuts and a softer look on layered hair. Spiral perms do not promote root lift so be sure to discuss this with your client. You should aim to complete a medium-length spiral wind in one hour.

? Memory jogger

Why do you need to remove rods very carefully?

Why does neutraliser need to be removed completely from the hair?

What are fish hooks and how are they avoided?

What does after-perm care mean?

UNIT GH6

Plait and twist hair using basic techniques

Plaiting and twisting hair is a very skillful technique and requires a high degree of manual dexterity (being good at using your hands). A single plait can give either an innocent or sophisticated look, depending on the style, whilst twists can be edgy and dramatic, completely changing the client's look. Both plaiting and twisting techniques can offer your clients something a little different, whether for everyday wear or a glamorous evening look. The techniques require patience and practice to perfect but you will then be able to offer them in addition to classic salon services, such as chemical treatments, cutting and styling.

This unit is about using basic plaiting and twisting techniques following the instructions of the stylist and is suitable for those working with Caucasian and Asian hair types. This unit applies for hairdressing students working in hairdressing and barbering salons.

In this unit you will learn about:

- Types of plaiting and twisting
- Maintaining effective and safe methods of working when plaiting and twisting
- Plaiting and twisting hair.

Here are some key words you will meet in this unit:

Sprays – used to hold a style

Serums – oil-based products used to smooth the cuticle

Gels – used to keep hair in place and add shine

Multiple corn rows – lots of tiny scalp plaits

French plait – usually one main plait secured to the scalp

Two strand twists – tiny twists involving two strands of hair

Traction alopecia – excessive tension applied to the hair and scalp causing baldness

Asian hair – the hair shaft is round in shape, straight and/or coarse

Caucasian hair – the hair shaft is oval in shape and can be straight, wavy or curly

Tangle-free – hair which has been combed smooth and is free from knots or tugs

Texture – the way hair feels, determined by touch during the consultation

Types of plaiting and twisting

Plaits are formed by intertwining (weaving together) strands of hair to create patterns or even structures. Material other than hair, such as ribbons or hair extensions, can be incorporated into the plait to give a more interesting finished look. Twists are formed by twisting sections of hair around each other. Both plaiting and twisting can create very artistic, intricate and ornate hairstyles, involving techniques that are very specialised and take time to master.

Plaits and twists can be created on short, medium and long hair, on any hair type or texture and on both males and females. They can be small or large and formed either close to the scalp or in loose hanging sections, giving the hair movement.

Looks that can be achieved by plaiting and twisting

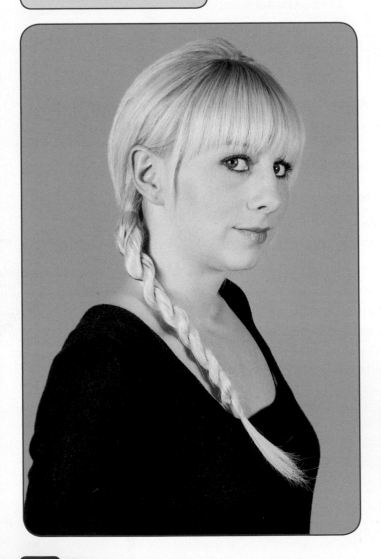

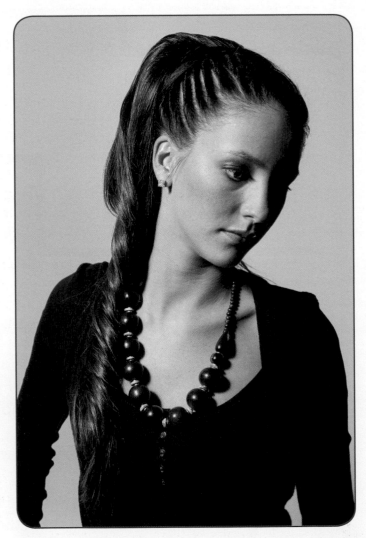

Before you can proceed with a plaiting or twisting service you will need to be sure the client's hair can cope with the tension (pulling) that will be applied. You will also need to consider what styles are likely to suit them by looking at their hair and facial characteristics. You will therefore need to think about the following:

- hair type
- hair length
- hair density
- hair elasticity
- head and face shape.

Always follow the instructions of your stylist.

Get up and go!

Get together with a colleague and think about how each other's hair type, length, density and elasticity, as well as face and head shape, will affect a plaiting or twisiting service. What style would each of you recommend to the other?

Considering hair types when plaiting and twisting

You will need to think about the type of hair your client has when carrying out plaiting and twisting techniques. Caucasian/European and Asian/Oriental hair types have important differences and you will need to be able to work with both. One of the major differences is texture, which will vary from client to client and may also vary within the same head of hair. Texture can be fine, medium or coarse, with fine hair having a small circumference and coarse hair having a large circumference. To determine the texture, run your fingers along the length of a single hair.

You also need to know about the dangers of applying too much pressure on the hair when plaiting and twisting. Hair that is excessively pulled can lead to a painful and irritable scalp, as well as hair breakage. If this pulling, or tension, continues the client may suffer from what is known as 'traction alopecia', where the hair is pulled from the scalp due to excessive tension, leaving a bald area. This area will remain bald until new hair grows back through – it can be a month before you see only 1.25cm of new hair.

Memory jogger

What types of things should you consider before carrying out a plaiting or twisting service?

How can Caucasian/European and Asian/Oriental hair differ?

What are the potential consequences of excessive tension on the hair and scalp?

Get up and go!

Find out about the different types of equipment that are used to create plaited and twisted styles. Don't forget about things like coloured hair pieces and hair ornaments that can be added.

Maintaining effective and safe methods of working when plaiting and twisting (I)

Protecting the client

Your client must be protected with clean towels, gown and waterproof cape. If your client is having colour added to their hair as part of the plaiting or twisting service, you may need to use particular towels intended for colouring. Remember that it is very important your client's clothes are adequately covered and protected during a colouring service.

Personal protective equipment (PPE)

Remember to wear suitable PPE when carrying out a plaiting or twisting service, particularly if you are using coloured sprays or gels. Gloves will protect your hands from these irritants, which can cause dermatitis.

Preparing the client for shampooing

Your client may need to have their hair shampooed before the plaiting or twisting service can be carried out. This may be due to a build up of styling products or perhaps the client's hair is excessively oily. Before shampooing, you will need to comb through the client's hair. Remove tangles carefully to avoid causing the client any discomfort. Check the client's scalp with the stylist, looking for any cuts or irritated areas which may need special attention. You will also need to discuss with the stylist the correct shampoo to use, which may be a clarifying shampoo that removes all previous products and leaves the hair in its most natural state.

Positioning the client and checking your own posture

As you prepare the client for the plaiting or twisting service, ask them whether or not they will need to move from the chair for any reason. The service may take an hour or two and so it is a good idea to find out if they have any physical needs you should be aware of. If they do need to get up and stretch or walk about during the service, you may like to offer them the opportunity to do so before you start any particularly tricky parts. Remember also to offer the client refreshments or a magazine before and regularly during the service.

As you will be working on the client for a long time, it is important to be aware of your own comfort. You should stand with straight legs and your feet slightly apart to maintain your balance. Keep your shoulders relaxed too. Taking these simple steps will help minimise your risk of developing injury and fatigue.

>> Get up and go!

What products does your salon offer that can be used to add colour to your client's hair as part of a plaited or twisted style? Should they be used on wet hair or dry hair? Do they require any processing time? Discuss your findings with your assessor.

Keeping your work area clean and tidy

It is essential that you keep your work area clean and tidy during the service. This will ensure the service runs smoothly and also gives a professional image to the client. Position tools and equipment for ease of use and prepare the trolley with all of the resources you will need for plaiting or twisting, ensuring they are clean and in good condition.

Preparing the resources for plaiting and twisting

You will need to prepare a trolley with the following items:

- client record card
- clean towels (of the appropriate colours)
- gloves
- apron
- selection of combs
- old hairdressing scissors
- extension hair (if required)
- soft bristled brush
- section clips
- aftercare products
- aftercare sheet/card.

All resources must be cleaned or sterilised after every use. This will help to minimise the risk of cross-infection.

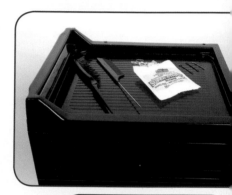

A trolley containing some equipment for plaiting and twisting

Maintaining effective and safe methods of working when plaiting and twisting (2)

Minimise the risk of damage to tools

The hairdressing profession relies on good quality, safe tools and equipment in good working order. Always do your best to look after your own tools and equipment and the salon's property. Before using, make sure items are safe and fit for their purpose, reporting any faults to the appropriate person.

Reducing product wastage

Before using any product, always read the manufacturer's instructions and discuss the instructions with the stylist. If you need to prepare a product, remember to prepare only the amount you need just before it is to be used. This will help to reduce wastage. If extra product is required, it is more cost-effective to make it freshly as you need it.

Reducing the risk of cross-infection

Reduce the risk of cross-infection by being alert to any signs of infection and covering any open wounds or cuts with a suitable waterproof dressing. Report any personal infection or infestation to the appropriate member of staff. Always practise good standards of personal hygiene and wear clean, well-pressed clothes every day. Clients who have an open cut or wound must be treated with particular care. Seek advice from the stylist or your assessor and find out if barrier cream would be appropriate on this occasion. The situation may require your client to return for the service once the open wound has healed.

All tools and equipment used during the service must be cleaned in the appropriate way. Make sure you are familiar with how to clean or sterilise everything you have used, including brushes, combs, section clips, gowns and towels. This will reduce the risk of cross-infection and ensure tools and equipment are kept in good condition.

>> **Get up and go!**

Discuss with a colleague what a commercially acceptable timeframe for plaiting and twisting hair is. Are these services listed on your salon price list? How much do they cost? Does your salon sell any products associated with plaiting and twisting? If so, what are they, how are they applied and how long do they last?

Reducing the risk of harm or injury to yourself, your colleagues and clients

Always keep a look out for hazards or risks which may arise during the course of the day. Clear away used product bottles and used materials such as bowls and cotton wool. Keep the floor clear from trailing cables, towels, gowns and cut hair, as well as items belonging to clients such as handbags, shopping bags, walking sticks and pushchairs. This will help to minimise the risk of any accidents occurring.

Removing plaits or twists

Depending on what style your client has gone for, they may need to come back to the salon to have their plaits or twists professionally removed. They may want to do it themselves, but inform them that it can be very time-consuming. You should discuss with the client a suitable timeframe to come back to the salon for a check-up appointment, which could be, say, two months after the plaits or twists were put in. Remember, the removal process must be costed as part of the salon's services and should appear on the price list. You should aim to remove a complete set of plaits or twists from short to medium-length hair in less than one hour.

? **Memory jogger**

What should you do if you find that a tool or piece of equipment is broken?

Why is it more cost-effective to make up products as you need them?

What might happen if the salon is left to become cluttered with used resources and items belonging to clients?

Plaiting and twisting hair (I)

Plaiting techniques – French plait

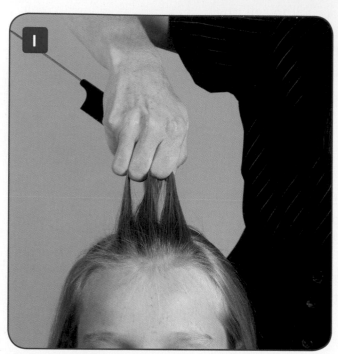

Correctly gown the client. Take the first section across the front hairline and divide into three strands

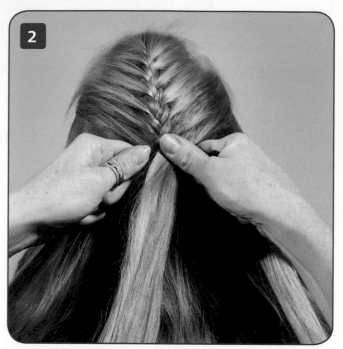

Cross the right hand section over into the centre, then cross the left hand section into the centre

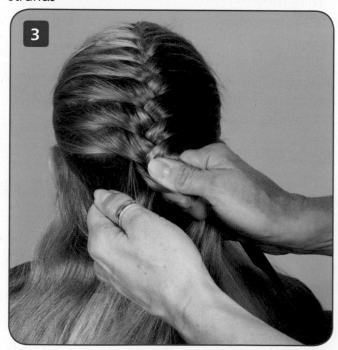

Pick up more hair from the sides as you work along the top of the head, keeping the hair taut. Smooth each section as you work from the front hairline section

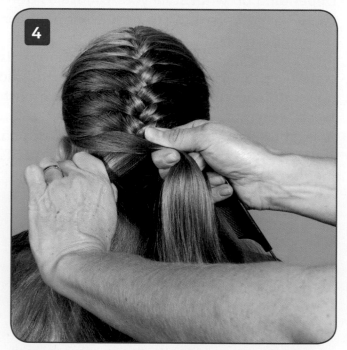

Keep the hair close to the client's scalp and the tension even as you continue to work towards the crown

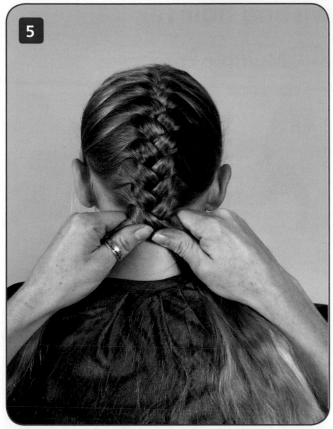

5

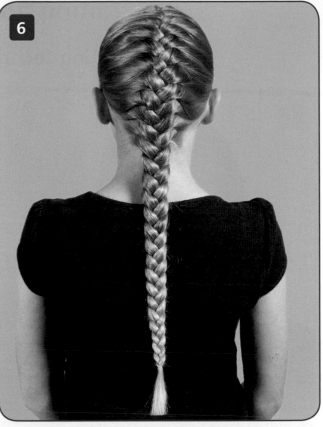

6

Continue to plait down the hair length and secure the free ends with a covered band or ribbon

The completed scalp plait secured to the head

Best practice for plaiting and twisting

- Always think about your client's comfort. Are they coping with any discomfort? Do you need to stop and reduce the tension?

- Neat sections and partings are crucial to the success of a style created by plaiting and twisting. They will also increase the lifespan of the hairstyle.

- Another important factor is even tension. You will have to reach a balance between applying enough tension to create the style and not causing your client too much discomfort or even hair breakage. You will soon learn to adjust the tension of plaits or twists to suit both the style and the client.

- Sections of hair not being worked on need to be held out of the way. Use section clips or butterfly clips and bring down only the amount of hair you need to work on.

- Apply suitable products as necessary during the service, taking care to follow manufacturers' and the stylist's instructions. The types of product you may need include sprays, serums and gels, which will help maintain the life of the hairstyle and give a professional finish.

Sharpen up!

List the different ways in which you can secure the client's hair when you have finished plaiting or twisting it.

Memory jogger

How do you secure the hair not being worked?

What will help make for a successful head of twists and plaiting?

How often should you check the client's comfort?

Plaiting and twisting hair (2)

Plaiting techniques – Multiple corn rows

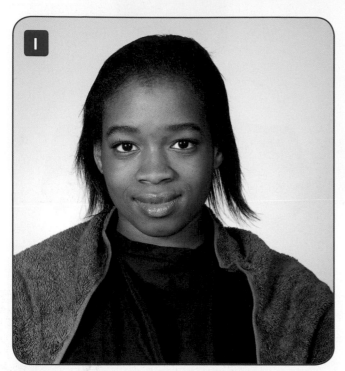

Correctly gown your client and, after your consultation, begin to section the hair

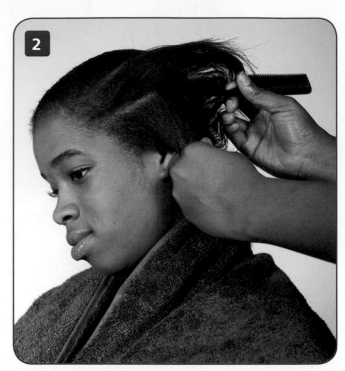

Begin sectioning at the sides

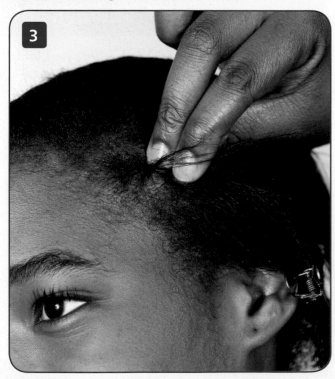

Form a small plait at the sides of the head

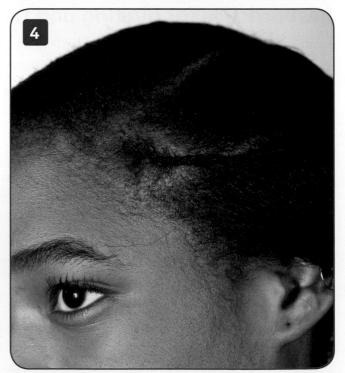

Work from the front hairline towards the nape area forming small neat plaits

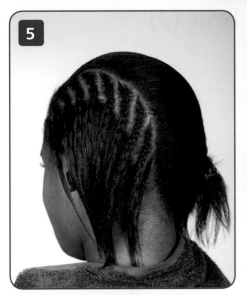

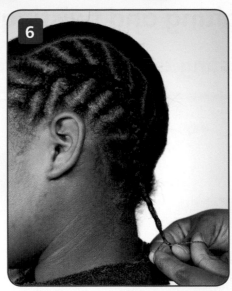

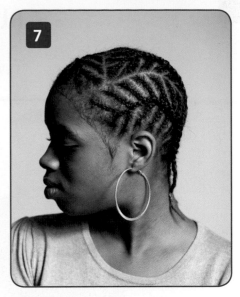

Plait the longer lengths together, working from the front through to the napes

The completed corn rows seen from the side

The finished look

Traction alopecia

Excessive tension (pulling) on the hair may lead to traction alopecia where the hair comes away from the scalp leaving bald areas. You will need to be alert for signs of this during a plaiting or twisting service. Look for:

- a sore/sensitive scalp
- weeping/pus at the roots
- a reduced amount of hair in an area.

Should traction alopecia occur, the area should be looked after with great care as any open sores may lead to an infection. Wearing plaits and twists continuously or regularly can lead to traction alopecia and so is not recommended. If your client becomes concerned, they should return to the salon for professional removal of the plaits or twists.

Any sign of alopecia needs to be recorded on your client's record card, noting the location of affected areas. Talk to your client about why this has happened and speak to your stylist about advice you can give to help improve the condition of their scalp.

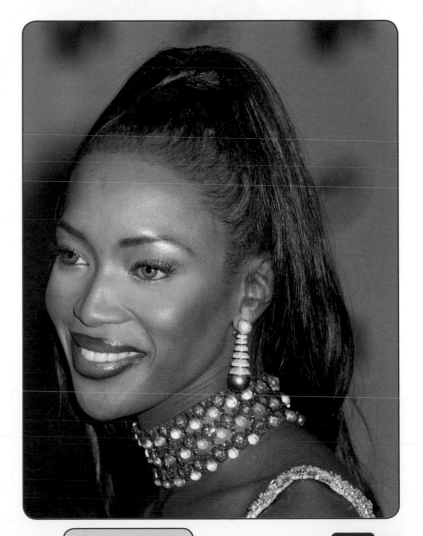

Traction alopecia

Plaiting and twisting hair (3)

Twisting techniques

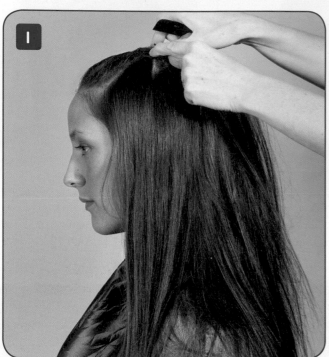

Prepare the client for the twisting service and begin to section the hair

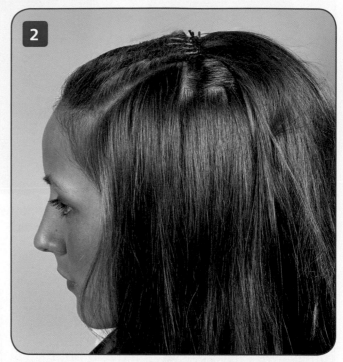

Take fine sections and twist the hair from the front hairline working back towards the crown

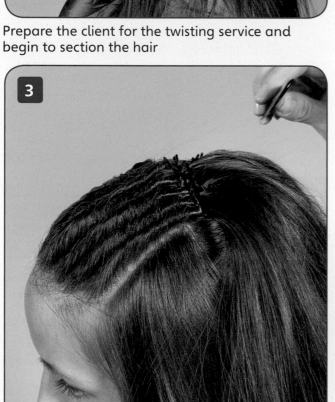

Secure the sections with hair grips as you work

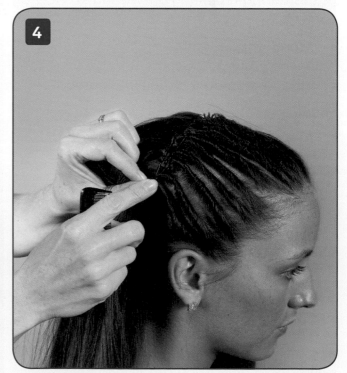

Work down either side starting at the top of the client's head each time

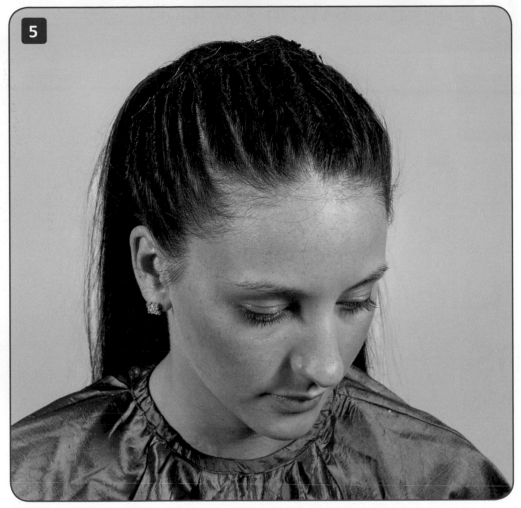

5

The completed look

Get ahead

Aftercare is a very important part of any hairdressing service. Clients who are well looked after are more likely to return to your salon rather than go somewhere else. Create an aftercare sheet or card for clients who have received a plaiting or twisting service. Remember to include basic details such as the salon's name and contact details, as well as your name and some advice on how they can look after their hairstyle at home. You could make this information into a list of 'dos and don'ts', for example.

Aftercare

You can start to advise your client on how to look after their plaits or twists as soon as you start the service. If it is a style that is meant to be worn for more than a day or two, you should advise your client how to keep their hair clean. Shampooing is still possible but they should not rub their hair vigorously, and plaits should be washed in the direction of the plait. Suitable oils and moisturisers can also be applied to the hair in order to protect it and add shine. These measures should minimise tangles and prolong the style.

You will need to advise the client how long they can wear their hair in plaits or twists before they should have them removed so as to prevent traction alopecia. Finally, be knowledgeable about the retail products in your salon and give the client helpful advice about the most appropriate products for their hair and style. Aftercare is part of professional client care and completes the plaiting or twisting service.

Memory jogger

How often should the client return for a consultation?

How soon do you start to advise your client on how to care for their new hairstyle?

Is it possible to shampoo hair with hair extensions?

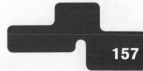

UNIT GH7

Remove hair extensions

Anne Veck, photographer: Clark Wiseman

Hair extensions can completely transform a client's look: short hair can be replaced by long flowing locks, and volume, texture, colour and curls can be added in no time at all. Hair extensions can be funky and wild or serious and sophisticated. They can be added for fun and fashion or to help a client regain their hairstyle because of thinning hair. With an increasing demand for hair extensions it is very beneficial to be able to offer your clients this service in your salon.

In this unit, you will learn how to remove hair extensions following the instructions of a stylist. You will need to be able to use a number of tools and products in order to do this effectively and safely. The work involved will be carried out under the supervision of the relevant person, such as the stylist or assessor. This unit applies to hairdressing students working in hairdressing and barbering salons and is suitable for those working with Caucasian and Asian hair types.

In this unit you will learn about:

- Maintaining effective and safe methods of working when removing hair extensions
- Removing hair extensions.

Here are some key words you will meet in this unit:

Tension – pressure applied to the hair and scalp by excessive pulling

Seal breaker – implement used to assist with removal of hair extensions

Traction alopecia – excessive tension applied to the hair and scalp causing baldness

Extensions – additional hair applied to natural hair to offer length, texture, volume and colour

Asian hair – the hair shaft is round in shape, straight and/or coarse

Caucasian hair – the hair shaft is oval in shape and can be straight, wavy or curly

Cuticle – outer layer of the hair shaft

Surface conditioner – conditioner which coats the outer layer of the hair shaft

Texture – the way hair feels, determined by touch during the consultation

Tangle-free – hair which has been combed smooth and is free from knots or tugs

Fatigue – weary; exhausted from over work or adopting a poor posture

Maintaining effective and safe methods of working when using hair extensions (I)

Why have hair extensions?

Hair extensions are either natural human hair or man-made synthetic hair fibres. They can be applied either by using heated equipment to seal the extensions to hair (hot hair extension systems) or by using other methods to seal the extensions (cold hair extensions). Cold systems can be less damaging to the hair than hot systems. A client may consider asking for hair extensions for the following reasons.

- If their hair is thin or thinning.
- To increase the length of their hair.
- To add volume.
- To add different colours without committing.
- To add curls or straightness.

>> **Get up and go!**

You could try to interest clients in hair extensions by wearing them in your own hair. Try wearing some different textures, lengths and colours in your hair and take notice of the comments your clients make. Talk to them about the advantages of wearing extensions and show them some suitable styles.

Considering hair types when adding extensions

As you have learned, Caucasian/European and Asian/Oriental hair does differ due to the shape of the hair shaft, with Caucasian hair having an oval cross-section and Asian hair having a round cross-section. Hair can also be coarse, medium or fine. You will need to find out what type of hair your client has for the hair extension service to be successful.

You also need to be aware of the dangers of applying too much pressure on the hair when placing hair extensions. Hair that is excessively pulled can lead to a painful and irritable scalp, as well as hair breakage. If this pulling, or tension, continues the client may suffer from what is known as 'traction alopecia', where the hair is pulled from the scalp due to excessive tension, leaving a bald area. This area will remain bald until new hair grows back through – it can be a month before you see only 1.25cm of new hair.

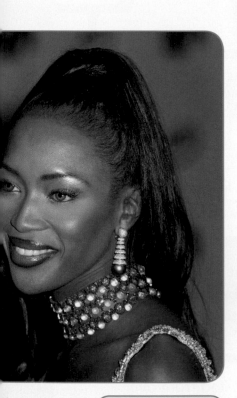

Traction alopecia

Protecting the client and yourself

Protect the client's clothing with the appropriate towel, gown and waterproof cape. For your own protection, remember to wear personal protective equipment (PPE) when working with clients who are receiving a hair extension service. Your hands and clothing must be protected at all times. Wear the right type of gloves and apron when using hair extension removal products as they can burn through certain types of plastic.

Preparing the client for shampooing

You will need to comb through the client's hair to remove any tangles before shampooing. Use this time to check the client's scalp for cuts or irritated areas with the stylist. You will also need to discuss with the stylist the correct shampoo to use, which will probably be a clarifying shampoo that will remove all traces of product and leave the hair in its most natural state. Now might be a good time to advise the client not to shampoo their hair again for at least two days after the service. This is to give the hair extensions time to fully adhere to the hair shafts, allowing them to set properly.

Positioning the client and checking your own posture

As you prepare the client for the hair extension removal service, ask them whether or not they will need to move from the chair for any reason. The service may take several hours and so it is a good idea to find out if they have any physical needs you should be aware of. If they do need to get up and stretch or walk about during the service, you may like to offer them the opportunity to do so before you start any particularly tricky parts. Remember also to offer the client refreshments or a magazine before and regularly during the service.

As you will be working on the client for a long time, it is important to be aware of your own comfort. You should stand with straight legs and your feet slightly apart to maintain your balance. Keep your shoulders relaxed too. Taking these simple steps will help minimise your risk of developing injury and fatigue.

> **» Get up and go!**
>
> Because hair extension removal products 'melt' the bonds that hold the extensions in place, they can also melt other plastics that they come into contact with. Think about the materials and tools you use on a daily basis in the salon that are made from plastic. How can they be protected from unnecessary damage? Discuss your thoughts with your assessor.

> **? Memory jogger**
>
> Why might a client request hair extensions?
>
> What causes traction alopecia?
>
> Why must you make sure you are wearing the correct type of PPE when handling hair extension removal products?

> **» Get up and go!**
>
> Think about the concerns usually experienced by clients when they have their hair extensions removed. What might they be worried about? How can you reassure them? Talk through your thoughts with your assessor.

Maintaining effective and safe methods of working when removing hair extensions (2)

Keeping your work area clean and tidy

It is essential to keep your work area clean and tidy during the service. This will ensure the service runs smoothly and also presents a professional image to the client. Position tools and equipment for ease of use and prepare the trolley with all the resources you will need for removing hair extensions, ensuring they are clean and in good condition.

Working safely with hair extension products and tools

As with any product you use in the salon, always read the manufacturer's instructions and check with the stylist before using. Only make up the amount you need just before you need to use it. Some of the tools used when working with hair extensions, such as straighteners and the hot-bond hair extension system, often reach very high temperatures. Take great care when using these items to minimise the risk of accidents or injury.

Reducing the risk of cross-infection

Reduce the risk of cross-infection by being alert to any signs of infection and covering any open wounds or cuts with a suitable waterproof dressing. Report any personal infection or infestation to the appropriate member of staff. Always practise good standards of personal hygiene and wear clean, well-pressed clothes every day. Clients who have an open cut or wound must be treated with particular care. Seek advice from the stylist or your assessor and find out if barrier cream would be appropriate on this occasion. The situation may require your client to return for the service once the open wound has healed.

All tools and equipment used during the service must be cleaned in the appropriate way. Make sure you are familiar with how to clean or sterilise everything you have used, including brushes, combs, section clips, gowns and towels. You will also need to clean the applicator gun with the recommended cleaning product. This will reduce the risk of cross-infection and ensure tools and equipment are kept in good condition.

Reducing the risk of harm or injury to yourself, your colleagues and clients

Always keep a look out for hazards or risks which may arise during the course of the day. Clear away used product bottles and used materials

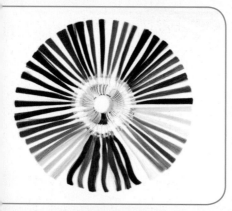

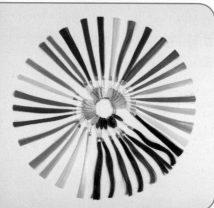

Hair extensions are available in different lengths and colours

such as bowls and cotton wool. Keep the floor clear from trailing cables, towels, gowns and cut hair, as well as items belonging to clients such as handbags, shopping bags, walking sticks and pushchairs. This will help to minimise the risk of any accidents occurring.

Skin and suitability tests

A skin test should be carried out before the hair extension service is carried out. The gum-based products used in a cold hair extension system come into contact with the client's scalp, so sensitivity and allergy to these products must be tested. The test is carried out by applying a small amount of the product to the client's skin or by applying a hair extension using the product.

A suitability test allows the stylist to make sure the client's hair is suitable for the hair extension service. The stylist will also tell the client what is involved with looking after extensions and ask whether they can do this. Between three and five extensions my be placed in the hair, for an agreed fee, and then the client will return to the salon for a check-up, which will determine suitability in terms of:

- Is the hair strong enough to hold extensions for three months?
- Has there been any hair breakage?
- Are there are signs of scalp irritation?
- Does the client fully understand how to care for their extensions?

The results of any test must always be recorded on the client's record card.

Preparing the resources for applying or removing hair extensions

You will need to prepare a trolley for the stylist with the following items:

- client record card
- clean towels
- barrier cream
- gloves
- apron
- selection of combs
- old hairdressing scissors
- mixing mat[1]
- extension hair[1]
- bonding gun[1]
- resin sticks[1]

- heatproof drip mat[1]
- soft-bristled brush
- section clips
- removal tools[2]
- scalp protectors
- aftercare products and advice card/sheet
- cotton wool
- removal solutions
- hair dryer.

[1] For extension application
[2] For extension removal

All resources must be cleaned or sterilised after every use. This will help to minimise the risk of cross-infection.

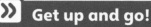

Get up and go!

Find out how to prepare the hair extensions used in your salon by reading the manufacturer's instructions. Discuss the result, and how you found following the instructions, with a senior colleague.

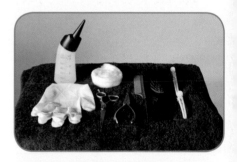

A trolley prepared for applying or removing hair extensions

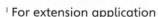

Memory jogger

Why is it important to work in a clean and tidy salon?

What does a suitability test involve and why is it carried out?

Name as many items as you can that are needed for a hair extension application service.

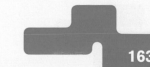

Removing hair extensions (I)

Before the appointment

When you have a client booked in to have their hair extensions removed, you will have to think about how long the extensions have been in the hair. It is recommended that hair extensions remain in place for no more than three months, but your client could be having them removed before or after this time. Hair grows about 1.25cm each month and the amount of growth since having the extensions applied can affect the removal service – extensions that have been in place for more than three months can be uncomfortable to remove. You might want to ask the client to apply conditioner to the bonds the night before their appointment, which will help break down the plastic resin, making the removal a little easier.

Preparing for the service

When your client is being prepared for the removal service, let them know it may feel like they are losing a lot of their hair as the extensions are removed. However, this hair loss will just be the hair they would have naturally shed over the time period they had the extensions. The client should also be made aware how long the service will take. Depending on the type of hair extensions they have, it may take between 30 minutes and three hours.

You will need to prepare a trolley for the extension removal service. Items you will need in addition to those listed on page 163 are:

- seal breakers
- removal products
- cotton wool pads
- hairdryer
- seam releasers.

Make sure you wear suitable personal protective equipment throughout the service, to include gloves and an apron. Remember: hair extension removal products can be dangerous if you are not properly protected.

Removing hair extensions as instructed by your stylist

First, you will need to separate the bonds one by one to make sure they have not become tangled together. You can then brush through the client's hair with a soft-bristled brush, working from the points of the hair through to the roots, being careful not to damage the natural hair.

Take care not to apply too much tension whilst brushing through the roots as this may irritate the scalp.

The removal process for most extension systems will be similar to the ones described below but you should always check the manufacturer's instructions.

Removing hot hair extension systems

Section the client's hair and start the removal process on the hairline around the nape. Place a cotton wool pad underneath the hair extension bond and apply the removal solution, allowing it to penetrate the bond completely for the recommended time. This will soften the plastic bond, allowing the extension to be gently pulled away from the client's hair. Seal breakers may be needed before or after applying the removal solution, but this is dependent on the manufacturer's instructions.

Removing cold hair extension systems

Removing cold hair extensions follows a similar process to that described for hot hair extensions, except that the heat from a handheld hairdryer is used to activate the removal solution.

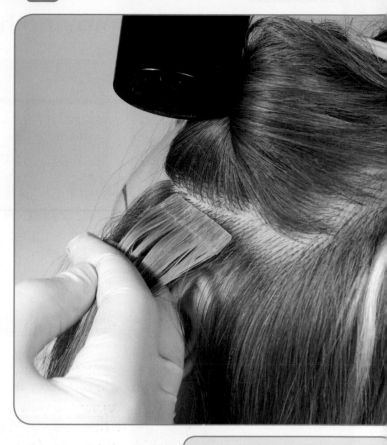

Using a hairdryer to speed up the removal of cold hair extensions

---

» Get up and go!

Why do you think a cotton wool pad is placed underneath the bond before applying the removal solution? Think about what the chemical does. Discuss your thoughts with your assessor.

? Memory jogger

What is the recommended maximum time for wearing hair extensions?

Why might some of the client's hair come away with the hair extensions?

Why is a hairdryer used when removing some cold hair extensions?

Why is it important to check the client's hair for any stray hair extensions?

Check all hair extensions have been removed

Check each section as you work through your client's hair, making sure you have removed all of the hair extensions. Extensions can be quite small and easily missed when working amongst a mass of hair. When all the extensions have been removed, comb through each section gently, working from point to root. The stylist will need to check all the extensions have been removed, and when they are satisfied, your client is ready for the next part of the service.

Removing hair extensions (2)

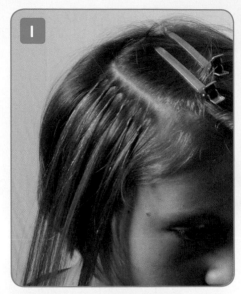

1 Prepare the trolley containing the tools and equipment needed for removing hair extensions

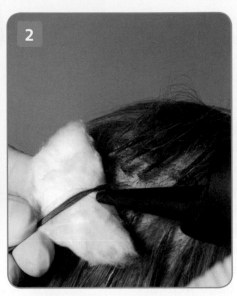

2 Wearing gloves to avoid any irritation, apply removal solution to soften the bond

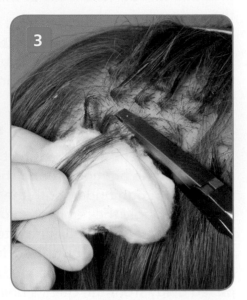

3 Break the bond with the seal breakers

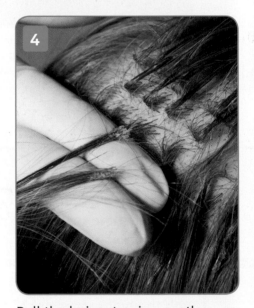

4 Pull the hair extension gently away from the scalp

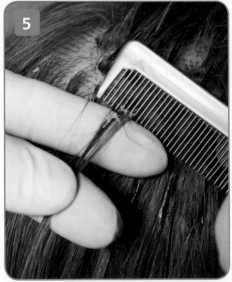

5 Use a fine tooth comb to remove excess softened glue

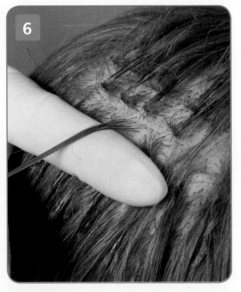

6 Continue to remove the remaining extensions

Best practice for removing hair extensions

- Always use products and equipment in line with the manufacturer's and stylist's instructions. Make sure you have understood any instructions given to you. If you are ever unsure, double check.

- Always use tools and equipment for their intended purpose and make sure you know how to use them properly. You will then be able to use them effectively and minimise any damage to your client's hair.

- Keep in mind the client's comfort throughout the service. Regularly check their position and ask them if they need to move or stand up.

- Gel or conditioner can be used to protect the client's own hair when applying removal solution to the extensions.

- Make sure the removal solution doesn't run onto your client's face or clothes.

> **» Get up and go!**
>
> Discuss with a colleague what a commercially acceptable timeframe is for removing hair extensions. Does this service appear on your salon price list?

Removing hair extensions can be very uncomfortable or even painful for the client if it is not done correctly. The removal solution can irritate and damage skin and clothes so be especially careful when applying it. Take particular care around the eyes and consider using barrier cream around the hairline to prevent any solution running into the client's eyes. Always work in a well ventilated area as the removal solution can be very strong smelling. If you have any concerns at all during the service, always refer to your stylist for advice.

Shampooing the client's hair

The next part of the service, after the extensions have been removed, is a shampoo. This will remove all traces of the removal solution and bonding product, as well as any conditioner or gel you used to protect the client's hair. After shampooing, towel-dry the client's hair and scalp and make sure they are clean and free from products and excess moisture. Take the client to the styling area and comb through their hair, leaving it tangle-free without damaging the hair or scalp. Your client's hair is now ready for the next service, which may be more hair extensions!

Aftercare

You will need to advise your client how best to look after their new hair extensions at home. Tell them about any suitable products your salon sells and give them advice on appropriate hair care. The client should not rub their hair when shampooing and conditioning as this will cause the extensions to tangle with the client's own hair. Good aftercare advice will help the client maintain their extensions, make them want to return to your salon next time, and completes the hair extension service.

Get ahead

Practise placing hair extensions on a male client. Applying a full head of hair extensions is time-consuming and requires neat and skilful work. You will need to think about a suitable colour, length, texture and style that are flattering to the client. Show your client some before and after photos and talk them through the process so they understand what will happen. Take some before and after photos of your client, as well as some photos of the process. You can use them to develop your portfolio, which can be used in your salon and at future interviews. You should aim to complete a full head of hair extensions on short to medium-length hair in less than four hours.

? Memory jogger

Why might you use gel or conditioner during the extension removal service?

Why shampoo the client's hair after removing extensions?

What aftercare advice could you give someone who has just had extensions applied?

UNIT GB1

Assist with shaving services

Anne Veck, photographer: David Howard

Barbering is one of the oldest hairdressing services. It is thought that the Egyptians were one of the first civilizations to develop barbering services, such as cutting hair and shaving. Many combs and cutting tools have been found during digs in various parts of Egypt. The cutting tools were sharpened flints, and the barbers would have met their clients in the street and carried out barbering services outside.

The word 'barber' is Latin and simply means 'beard'. Barbers used to carry out surgery as well as shaving services. Bandages stained with blood would be hung up to dry outside the barber's shop, and this is why barbers today sometimes have a red and white pole outside their business. The beard has long been a way of non-verbally communicating information such as the status and style of the wearer. A beard may tell you that the wearer is religious, wise or important, or it can simply be a way of saying, 'I am a man'. Facial hair styles change along with other fashions and trends but shaving services are always popular and in demand.

This unit is about the basic skills of shaving. The work involved will be carried out under the direction of the relevant person, such as the barber or assessor. This unit will apply for hairdressing students working in hairdressing and barbering salons.

In this unit you will learn about:

- Maintaining effective and safe methods of working when assisting with shaving services
- Preparing facial hair and skin for shaving services.

Here are some key words you will meet in this unit:

Lathering products – shaving creams and foams that are used as lubricants

Lubricant – a product which makes the surface of the skin slippery

Sharps – razors, scissors, needles, etc.

Astringents – products which have a stimulating effect on the skin

Contra-indication – an indication of the skin which would mean an alternative course of action

Barber – literally means 'beard'

Autoclave – sterilising system using moist heat

Barbicide – method of disinfecting tools in solution

Dermatitis – dry, itchy skin caused by an irritant

Effleurage – a stroking massage movement

Petrissage – a circular massage movement

Shaving brush – a small bristle brush used to apply lathering products

Maintaining effective and safe methods of working when assisting with shaving services (I)

Protecting the client

Your client must be protected with suitable and clean towels, gown and cape throughout the service. You will also need to have small pieces of cotton wool to hand to cover your client's eyes at certain times during the service. This is to protect the client's eyes from any product you may use or stray hair clippings when shaping the outline of the client's facial hair. It is important to regularly check your client's clothes are adequately covered and protected during shaving.

Personal protective equipment (PPE)

Remember to wear personal protective equipment (PPE) when assisting with shaving services. Your hands and clothing must be protected at all times. Dermatitis is a skin condition that makes your skin dry, sore and itchy. It is caused by irritants, such as chemicals in products, coming into contact with the skin. Use barrier cream or a good quality hand cream when working in the salon to help prevent your skin from drying out and to protect yourself from irritants. Gloves will prevent irritants from coming into contact with the skin. Gloves should also be worn when dealing with sharps and you will need to make sure the barber has a pair of gloves ready for their use. You will be working with sharp cutting and shaving tools and it is important to protect yourself properly.

 Sharpen up!

Does your salon or barber's have a towel colour system? If so, find out what colour towel you would use for a shave.

Positioning the client and checking your own posture

The client will sit in an adjustable barber's chair for the shaving service and you will need to adjust the elevation of the back of the chair to suit the barber who will be carrying out the service. Once you have

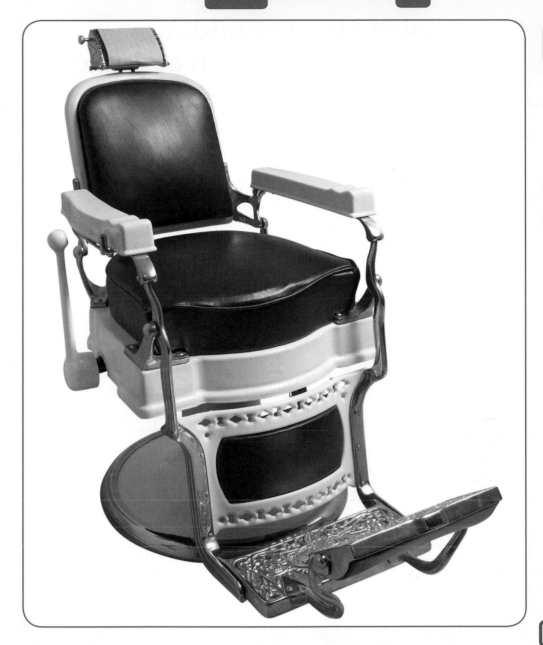

An adjustable barbering chair

adjusted the chair, make sure it is locked into position. Check your client's neck is positioned correctly in the curve of the neck rest and make sure they are comfortable. Ask if there are any areas they find easier or more difficult to shave. This information will help the barber and make the experience more comfortable for the client.

⟫ Get up and go!

Ask your barber if you can practise using the barbering chair. You need to be knowledgeable about how it operates and the benefits of using such a chair. Practise with a colleague.

❓ Memory jogger

What items can you use to protect your client during a shave?

Why should you wear suitable PPE when assisting with shaving services?

Why is the client's position and comfort important?

Maintaining effective and safe methods of working when assisting with shaving services (2)

Keeping your work area clean and tidy

It is essential to keep your work area clean and tidy during shaving services. Think about the tools, equipment and products you are going to need and make sure you have them to hand. Clear away anything that has been used and won't be needed again. This will ensure you don't waste time or keep your client waiting while you go back and forth getting things, or look for the things you need in a messy work area. Keeping your work area clean and tidy will enable you to work more effectively and it also helps keep your workplace safe.

Working safely with products

Before using any product, always read the manufacturer's instructions and discuss the instructions with the barber. Only use products for their intended purpose and wear appropriate PPE when handling if necessary. If you are asked to use a product, only prepare the amount you need just before it is to be used. This will help to reduce wastage. If extra product is required, it is more cost-effective to prepare the product as you need it.

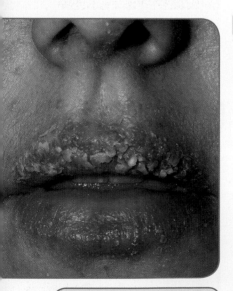

You must keep the work area clean and tidy

Impetigo is a bacterial skin infection

> **» Get up and go!**
>
> Find out how to prepare the various products used in your salon or barber's for lathering the skin. Read the manufacturer's instructions and then discuss them with the barber. Talk about your findings with a junior colleague.

Reducing the risk of cross-infection

Cross-infection is when an infection is passed from one person to another. You can take some very simple steps as you work to reduce the risk of this happening. Remember to always practise good personal hygiene and wear clean, well-pressed clothes. If you or any of your clients are showing signs of infection or infestation, you must report it straight away to a senior member of staff. They can then advise you what to do. If you have an open cut or wound, cover it with a suitable waterproof dressing. Clients with open cuts or wounds must be treated with particular care. Seek advice from the barber and ask if barrier cream would be appropriate at this stage. The situation may require your client to return once their wound has healed.

The two main infections you need to be aware of when assisting with shaving services are impetigo and barber's rash. Impetigo is a bacterial infection and can be recognised by yellow, crusty spots on the skin. Barber's rash is inflammation of the hair follicle, usually caused by unsterilised razors and shaving brushes. If you think the client has any kind of infection, promptly inform the barber.

You should also make sure you know how to use your salon's methods of sterilisation properly and ensure you always use clean tools and equipment on each new client. The main methods of sterilisation used in salons and barber's are:

- barbicide jars
- ultraviolet cabinets
- autoclaves.

All tools must be thoroughly cleaned with hot soapy water before being placed in any sterilisation equipment. Barbicide solution must be made up to the correct strength by reading the manufacturer's instructions and should be changed every day.

Ultraviolet cabinets use ultraviolet light to destroy bacteria, but as light is used, tools must be turned over so all sides are sterilised.

Autoclaves work like a pressure cooker and sterilise tools by heating them to high temperatures.

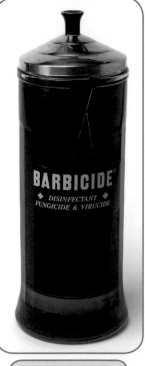

A jar of barbicide

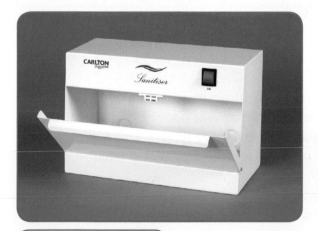

An ultraviolet cabinet

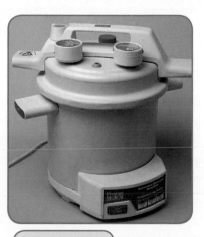

An autoclave

? Memory jogger

Why is it important to prepare for a shaving service by getting ready all the tools and products you will need?

What are the advantages of only making up products as you need them?

Describe what impetigo and barber's rash are.

What must you do to each piece of equipment before you use any method of sterilisation?

Maintaining effective and safe methods of working when assisting with shaving services (3)

Reducing the risk of harm or injury to yourself, your colleagues and clients

Always keep a look out for hazards or risks which may arise during the course of the day. Clear away used product bottles and used materials such as bowls, cotton wool and razors. Keep the floor clear from trailing cables, towels, gowns and cut hair, as well as items belonging to clients such as shopping bags, walking sticks and pushchairs. This will help to minimise the risk of any accidents occurring.

>> **Get up and go!**

Look at the different types of lighting in your salon or barber's. Do you have fluorescent tubes, spotlights or incandescent lights? Try to encourage your manager to go green and install energy-saving bulbs. They use up to 75% less electricity and last nearly ten times as long. Create a chart comparing the costs of each type of light along with their advantages and disadvantages. Show it to your manager and discuss how it might be more cost-effective and environmentally friendly to change the current lighting. Why might changing the lighting be costly at first but a good investment in the long run?

Re-ordering products

If the stock levels of a product are running low, remember to follow your salon's policy for re-ordering, which will probably involve telling the appropriate member of staff or writing it down. This will ensure you have sufficient products available, and also avoid having too much stock.

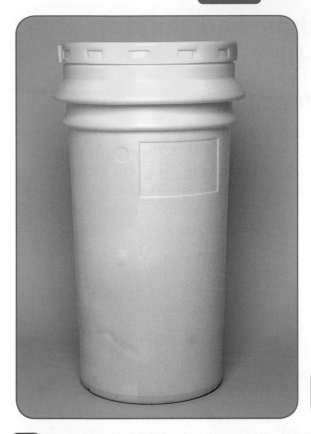

Used razor blades must be disposed of in a sharps bin

Disposal of waste

It is very important that you dispose of chemicals in the proper manner. Your salon or barber's must follow the Control of Substances Hazardous to Health (COSHH) Regulations and ensure products are disposed of in a safe and environmentally friendly way. Some salons have a specific basin for disposing of chemicals. Never pour chemicals down the sink in the salon's food and drink preparation area. Always flush them down the shampoo basin, followed by lots of cool water to make sure no smells or chemical waste linger round the basin.

Used razors must be placed in a sharps bin, which is then collected by a specialist refuse company. Waste also includes hair clippings, used cotton wool pads, disposable gowns and tissues. Make sure you dispose of these in line with COSHH and salon policy.

Preparing facial hair and skin for shaving services (I)

Preparing the client for shaving

Shaving is the art of removing facial hair entirely or creating shapes in it using either a manual razor or an electric razor. The overall purpose of shaving is to remove the unwanted hair from the client's face, leaving it in a desired style such as a beard or moustache, whilst also outlining neck hair and sideburns. The client needs to be consulted prior to the shave to find out what style they want.

Assessing the client's skin

Before carrying out a shaving service, the barber will assess the suitability of the client's skin, taking into consideration:

- existing skin conditions
- any cuts or abrasions
- facial skin features such as moles, scars or abnormalities of the surface of the skin
- facial piercings
- existing facial hair and its growth pattern
- shape and length of sideburns
- whether or not hot towels will be needed to soften the beard area prior to the shave.

A client prepared for a shaving service

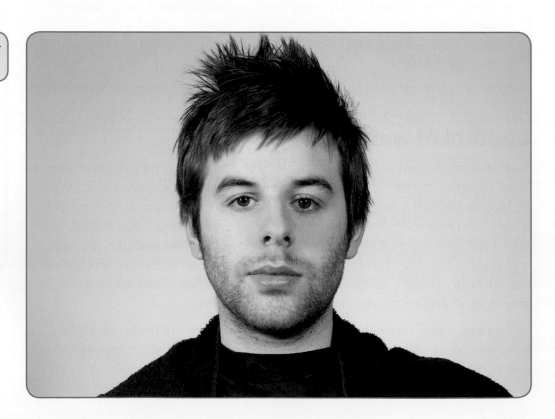

Resources for shaving

You will need to prepare a trolley for the barber with the following items:

- client record card
- clean towels (of the appropriate colours)
- apron
- gloves
- barrier cream
- cotton wool pads
- tissues
- plastic bowl
- pre-packed towels ready for steaming
- powder
- shaving foam/cream/gel/oils
- disposable styptic pencil
- shaving brushes
- barbicide jar
- cooling products
- aftershave
- moisturiser
- disposable razors.

>> **Get up and go!**

With a colleague, practise setting up a trolley for a shaving service. Check each other's trolleys for any missing items. Now set up a trolley for each other, but deliberately forget one item. See if you can spot what is missing.

Sharpen up!

A lot of equipment is needed to carry out a professional shaving service. Do you know what each item is used for, for example, do you know why a styptic pencil might be used?

Disposable razors are commonly used for shaving, but some barbers will use a traditional fixed blade razor (also know as a straight razor or 'cut-throat' razor). Fixed blade razors are sometimes not allowed to be used in salons and barber's because they can be dangerous and must be handled with extreme care. Find out if your local council permits their use and what regulations are in place regarding the use of sharps for professional barbering services. Present this information to your colleagues as part of your communication skills.

Preparing facial hair and skin for shaving services (2)

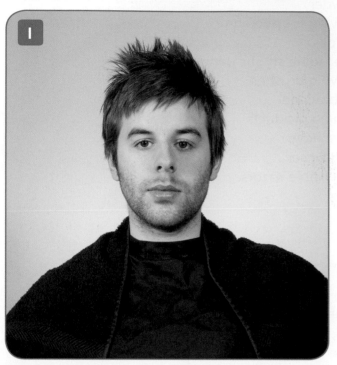

1

Correctly gown the client and carry out your consultation

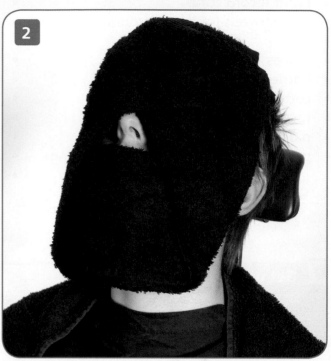

2

Place a hot towel around your client's face

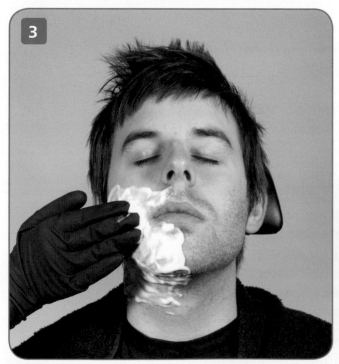

3

Begin to apply the lather

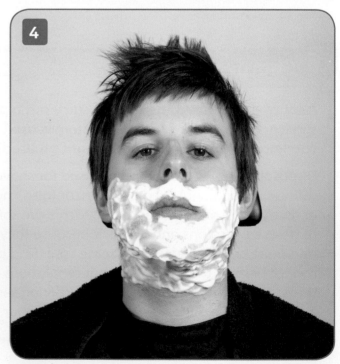

4

When your client is fully lathered the shave can begin

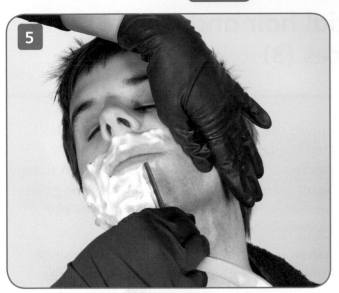

The barber will now carry out the shave

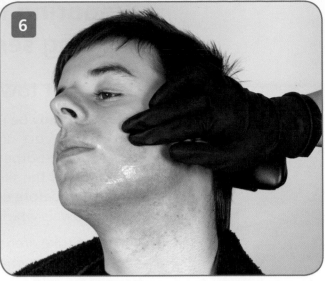

When the shave is complete, apply moisturisers to soothe and cool the skin

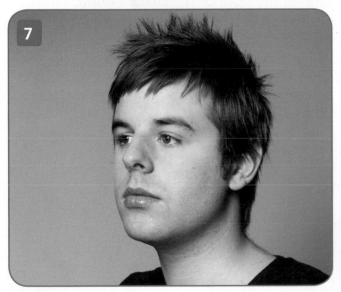

The finished look

 Sharpen up!

If you are male, you could try to interest clients in shaving services by wearing a moustache or beard at the salon/barber's. If you are female, you could enlist the help of a male colleague and help them try out different facial hair styles. Try this for a few weeks and take notice of comments clients make. Show them some of the different styles available and offer to assist them in trying a new look.

Preparing facial hair and skin for shaving services (3)

Using hot towels

Hot towels may be used during the shaving service to open up the pores on the face and soften the facial hair. This can make shaving easier for the barber and more comfortable for the client. A hot towel also cleanses the skin and can be relaxing for the client. Towels must be cleaned before each use. Some salons and barbers will use pre-packed towels which simply require steaming.

You must take great care when using hot towels as they can be hot enough to burn when freshly steamed. It is a good idea to practise handling a cold towel first to get your technique right before moving on to a hot towel. Wring out the towel until it is nearly dry, using a dry towel to help prevent burning yourself. Fold the towel to retain the heat and test its temperature on the back of the client's hand. Wrap the towel carefully around the client's face, leaving a space for his nose so he can breathe. Repeat this process two or three times and as you take the last towel off, begin immediately to lather the client's face.

A hot towel ready for the client

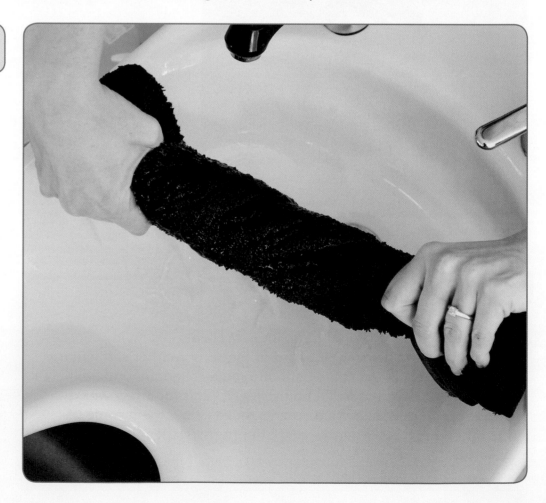

Lathering the client

Protect the client's eyes with cotton wool pads and ensure their neckline is protected with towels and tissues. Start applying lather under the chin, working in small circular movements moving upwards towards the left side of the face and then over to the right. Spread the bristles of the shaving brush out as you lather the top lip, being careful not to push the bristles inside the client's nose.

Work quickly and efficiently when lathering, making sure you cover only those parts of the face that are to be shaved. Lather must be applied evenly – not too thick or too thin. The purpose of lathering is to soften the hair and make the shave more comfortable for the client. If the hair is especially dense or strong, you may need to massage it into the facial hair with your hands, which will soften the hair further.

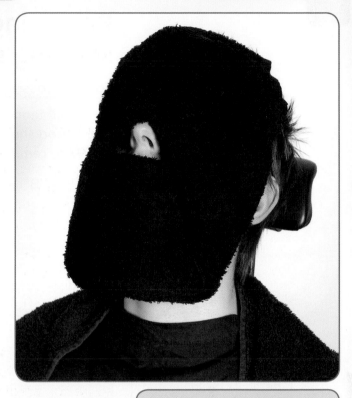

A hot towel will open the pores and soften the facial hair

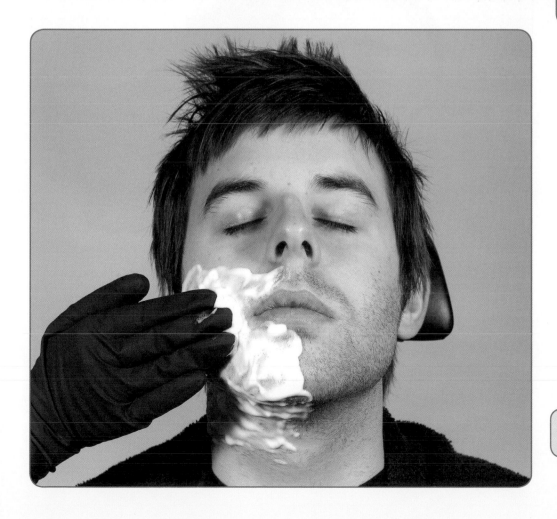

Lather being applied to the client

Preparing facial hair and skin for shaving services (4)

Facial massage movements

You have learned about three massage movements that are carried out during shampooing and conditioning hair (look back at pages 96–97 to remind yourself):

- effleurage
- rotary
- petrissage.

You can use effleurage and petrissage movements on the face during shaving services. The light, slow, stroking movement of effleurage will help distribute the lather, whilst the circular movement of petrissage will help soften the cuticles of the hair shafts.

> Facial massage can help distribute the lather and soften the hair

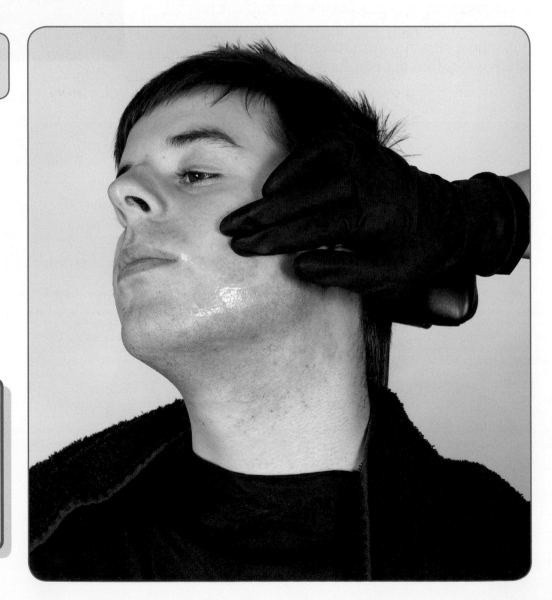

>> **Get up and go!**

Practise using facial massage movements on a colleague and ask for feedback regarding the pressure and timeliness of the massage.

Assisting further with the shave

After completing the application of the lather, you should inform the barber who will then start the shave. Be on hand during the shave as you may be needed to supply additional products or materials, or to apply more lather if it begins to dry out.

When the barber has finished the shave, you will need to apply hot or cold towels as required. Your client may have opted for hot towels, which can be relaxing and calming or, alternatively, they may enjoy the invigorating effects of a cold towel to give them a fresh, lively feeling. Leave the skin free from all products and excessive moisture by towel blotting. You can now analyse the skin with the barber to determine whether it is suitable to apply further products or give a face massage, checking with your client if they would like this. Shaving balms, which cool and moisturise the skin, and aftershaves, which stimulate the skin, are popular choices following a shave.

Should there be any problems during the service, report them immediately to the barber, who will advise you what to do. Common problems include bleeding after the shave, which can be controlled by applying pressure to the site of the blood with cotton wool. Make sure you are wearing gloves whilst doing this. A disposable styptic pencil or a little powder can also help with the bleeding.

Aftercare

Aftercare is an important part of the shaving service and could mean the difference between the client choosing to return or not. Give your client advice on when next to return for a shaving service and also when and how to use suitable exfoliating products. These will help remove dead skin cells from the surface layer of the skin and prevent hairs from growing into the skin.

> **⬆ Get ahead**
>
> Practise using a stencil, and design different styles into your client's hair. Use a training head in the early stages of your development, then progress to a client who you have consulted with, to create your own signature styles. Take photographs of your styles and build up a style book for use in the salon.

> **❓ Memory jogger**
>
> List three resources needed for shaving.
>
> What are the steps taken before the blade touches the client's skin?
>
> Why are hot towels used?
>
> Would preparation of an open razor include sterilising or lubricating?

> **≫ Get up and go!**
>
> Using paper and pencil, create some facial hair styles of your own. Think about styles that will suit different types of people. Now attempt to recreate your styles on a training head, progressing to a client. Take photographs of the results and build up a style book for use in your salon or barber's.

Index